THE PROCESS OF CULTURAL COMPETENCE IN THE DELIVERY OF HEALTHCARE SERVICES

The Journey Continues

J. CAMPINHA-BACOTE

Contents

Chapter 5

Chapter 6

Conclusion

Bibliography

Appendices & Figures

Scaling the Mountain

"When he took the time to
help the man up the mountain,
lo, he scaled it himself."
Tibetan Proverb

This Tibetan proverb serves as a metaphor for understanding how we are to *scale the mountain* of cultural competence. It is when we take the time to help others that we in turn tread our own personal path towards cultural competence. As healthcare professionals, we are considered the "helping profession." Ironically, as noted in this above quote, it is our patients and others who truly help us. We cannot afford to view our patients as difficult, non-compliant, or the less value-laden term, non-adherent. Instead they are to be viewed as helpers and cultural informants in our journey towards cultural competence in healthcare delivery.

Two of my most extraordinary cultural informants are my mother and father, to whom I dedicate this book. John W. Whitehead once said, "Children are living messages we send to a time we will not see." I can humbly say that it is the many messages that my parents gave me, during their life and in their death that has greatly enriched my worldview as I continue to scale the mountain of cultural competence. In this book, I share some of the lessons I have learned by my many cultural informants.

Cultural Competence: Making the Difference

*"When we lose the right to be different,
we lose the privilege to be free."*
Charles Evans Hughes

In responding to the current and projected demographic changes within the United States, healthcare professionals face the challenge of providing culturally responsive services to our ever-growing multicultural world. Cross, Bazron, Dennis & Isaac's (1989) groundbreaking definition of cultural competence has been the most widely accepted and utilized definition of cultural competence in health care. These authors characterize cultural competence as "a set of congruent behaviors, attitudes, and policies that come together in a system, agency, or amongst professionals and enables that system, agency, or those professionals to work effectively in cross-cultural situations" (p. iv).

Despite the many additional definitions of cultural competence since Cross' et al. (1989) definition, and the development of several models of care and service delivery efforts to meet the challenges of providing culturally responsive service, healthcare professionals continue to ask the question, "What does it mean to be a culturally competent healthcare professional?" To adequately address this question, we must first define the concept of culture.

Defining Culture

The literature is saturated with definitions of culture; however, Tylor's (1871) definition serves as the foundational definition of culture for this text. Tylor defines culture as "that complex and whole which includes knowledge, belief, art, morals, law, custom and any other capabilities and habits acquired by man as a member of a society

(p. 1). This definition was purposefully selected for it suggests a broad view of culture

which is not limited to looking at cultural groups in terms of ethnicity or nation of origin

only, but is inclusive of cultural groups that are based on religious affiliation, language,

physical size, gender, sexual orientation, age, disability (both physical and mental),

political orientation, socio-economic status, occupational status and geographical

location, to name a few. Using Tylor's definition of culture it becomes clear to see that

every person has more than a single cultural identity and belongs to several different

cultural groups.

The concept of culture and its relationship to health is critical to comprehend

when discussing cultural competence in healthcare delivery, for cultural values give an

individual a sense of direction and meaning to life. As eloquently stated by Leininger

(1967), "culture is tightly interwoven into the life of man and continuously pervades his

thinking, actions, feelings and particularly his health state."

Building the Case for Cultural Competence in Healthcare Delivery

The National Center for Cultural Competence (Cohen & Goode, 1999) identifies

six reasons why cultural competence is needed in health care:

1. Responding to current and projected demographic changes in the United States
2. Eliminating long-standing disparities in the health status of people of diverse racial, ethnic, and cultural backgrounds
3. Improving the quality of services and outcomes
4. Meeting legislative, regulatory, and accreditation mandates
5. To gain a competitive edge in the market place
6. To decrease the likelihood of liability/malpractice claims

To further build the case for cultural competence, there have been many appraisals of the Nation's health care and mental health delivery system revealing racial and ethnic disparities in health care. Two of these landmark reports include the Institute of Medicine's (IOM) publication entitled *Unequal Treatment: Confronting Racial and Ethnic Disparities in Health Care* (2003) and the 2001 Surgeon General's report on *Race, Culture and Ethnicity and Mental Health.*

The Institute of Medicine (IOM) report revealed that a large body of research supports the findings that racial and ethnic minorities in the United States receive lower quality health care than whites, even when insurance status, income, age and severity of condition are comparable (Smedley et al., 2002). Examples of health care disparities found in the IOM report note that minorities:

- are less likely to be given appropriate cardiac medications or to undergo bypass surgery;
- are less likely to receive kidney dialysis or transplants;
- are less likely to receive appropriate cancer diagnostic tests and treatments;
- are less likely to receive the most sophisticated treatments for HIV infections; and
- are more likely to receive some less desirable procedures, such as lower limb amputations for diabetes and other conditions.

Similarity, the Surgeon General's report on *Race, Culture and Ethnicity and Mental Health,* compellingly documents racial and ethnic disparities in mental heath care surrounding issues of misdiagnosis, underutilization, overrepresentation, and improper treatment (U.S. Department of Health and Human Services, 2001). These mental health disparities continue to surface with recent studies documenting racial and ethnic disparities in psychopharmacological treatment, resulting in minorities receiving mental health treatment that is not in concordance with recommended practices (Kuno &

Rothbard, 2002; Knudsen et al., 2007; Pi & Simpson, 2005; Snowden, 2004).

Specifically, Pi and Simpson (2005) noted differences in the prescribing patterns of second-generation antipsychotic drugs among Hispanics. In this study, Hispanics did not receive the newer, more effective second-generation antipsychotic agents as frequently as their non-Hispanic white counterparts. Not receiving such second-generation antipsychotic drugs increases the risk for tardive dyskinesia and extrapyramidal symptoms and may result in less clinical improvement. Explanations are multifaceted, however, there is evidence to believe that these racial and ethnic disparities are related to the lack of cultural competence among clinicians.

In 2000, the United States Department of Health and Human Services Office of Minority Health released national standards for the provision of culturally and linguistically appropriate services (CLAS) in health care (Appendix A). CLAS is a major document that has been helpful in providing healthcare professionals and healthcare organizations with guidelines for implementing culturally and linguistically competent care. These standards are intended to be used as a means to address and correct inequalities that exist in providing quality health care to culturally and ethnically diverse groups.

Summary

As demographic shifts translate into an ethnically diverse society, the concept of cultural competence has become a more increasingly common term in the United States (Jones et al., 2004, p. 283). There is compelling research and documentation supporting that the lack of cultural competence among healthcare professionals can result in poor health outcomes. The intent of this book is to provide healthcare professionals with a

12

culturally conscious approach to positively impact on the quality of healthcare services for *all* patients. This task will be accomplished by taking readers on a personal journey towards cultural competence in healthcare delivery. This journey will include examining **The Process of Cultural Competence in the Delivery of Healthcare Services** model and providing clinical application of this model's constructs of cultural desire, cultural awareness, cultural knowledge, cultural skill, and cultural encounters. After reading this book, it is my hope that you will be able to unequivocally answer the question, "What does it mean to be a culturally competent healthcare professional?"

Let The Journey Begin!

CHAPTER 1

The Process of Cultural Competence in the Delivery of Healthcare Services

"Adding wings to caterpillars does not create butterflies--
it creates awkward and dysfunctional caterpillars.
Butterflies are created through transformation."
Stephanie Marshall

The Process of Cultural Competence in the Delivery of Healthcare Services is a practice model of cultural competence in health care that defines **cultural competence as the ongoing process in which the healthcare professional continuously strives to achieve the ability and availability to work effectively within the cultural context of the patient (individual, family, community)** (Campinha-Bacote, 2003a). This model requires healthcare professionals to see themselves as *becoming* culturally competent rather than *being* culturally competent and involves the integration of cultural desire, cultural awareness, cultural knowledge, cultural skill and cultural encounters.

Development of the Model

My journey of cultural competence began in 1969 when I first experienced the challenges of being a Cape Verdean American in a world that classified individuals as either black or white. This experience brought me to a place of passion and interest in the area of cultural diversity. However, it wasn't until my professional experience in health care and mental health, several years later, that I blended my passion of culture and health care into the newly emerging field of cultural competence in health care.

I developed the prototype of my current model in 1991, when I initially identified the constructs of cultural awareness, cultural knowledge, cultural skill, and cultural encounters (Figure 1). In 1998 I revised this model by adding a fifth construct (cultural desire), modifying the pictorial representation of the model to reflect the interdependent relationship between the constructs, and expanding the definitions of the constructs to include new developments in the field of transcultural health care (Figure 2). After internalizing the newly developed construct of cultural desire, in 2002 I further revised my pictorial model to symbolically represent a volcano. Cultural competence is pictorially depicted as a volcano and symbolically, when cultural desire erupts, it gives forth the desire to "want to" enter into the process of becoming culturally competent by genuinely seeking cultural encounters, obtaining cultural knowledge, possessing the skill to conduct culturally sensitive assessments and being humble to the process of cultural awareness (Figure 3). I recognize that there are dynamic changes in this field and I will continue to be open to further revisions of my model.

Knowledge Antecedents

The Process of Cultural Competence in the Delivery of Healthcare Services model blends the fields of transcultural nursing, transcultural medicine, medical anthropology, cross-cultural psychology, theology and hospital administration by drawing upon the works of Leininger (1978), Kleinman (1980), Pederson (1988), Law (1993), Woods (1995) and Chapman (2005).

A Culturally Competent Model of Care

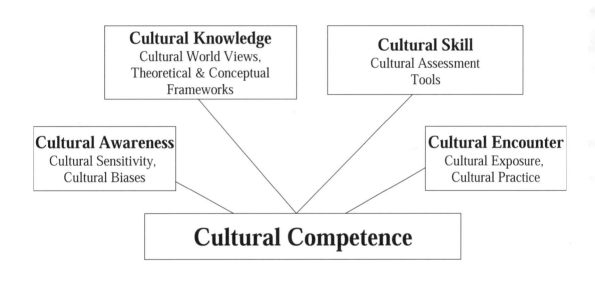

Figure 1

The Process of Cultural Competence in the Delivery of Healthcare Services

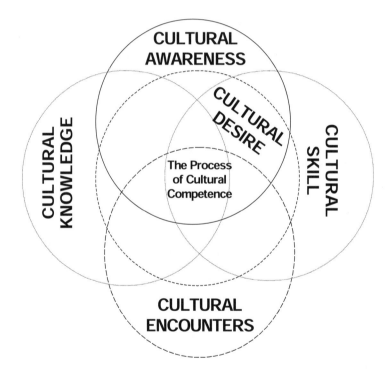

Figure 2

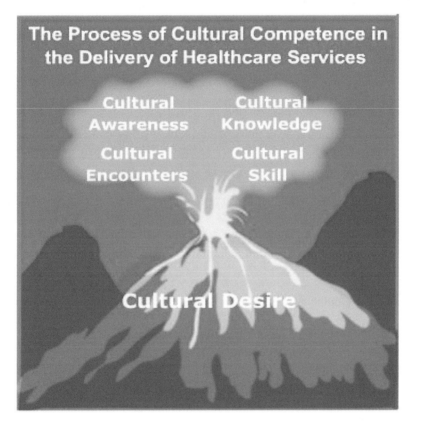

Figure 3

Assumptions of the Model

1. Cultural competence is a process, not an event; a journey, not a destination; dynamic, not static; and involves the paradox of knowing (the more you think you know; the more you really do not know; the more you think you do not know; the more you really know).

2. The process of cultural competence consists of five inter-related constructs: cultural desire, cultural awareness, cultural knowledge, cultural skill and cultural encounters.

3. The spiritual and pivotal construct of cultural competence is cultural desire.

4. There is variation within cultural groups as well as across cultural groups (intra-cultural variation).

5. Cultural competence is an essential component in rendering effective and culturally responsive care to all clients.

6. All encounters are cultural and sacred encounters.

Summary

The Process of Cultural Competence in the Delivery of Healthcare Services is a practice model of cultural competence in healthcare delivery that involves the conscious integration of cultural desire, cultural awareness, cultural knowledge, cultural skill and cultural encounters. To more fully understand this practice model, each of the model's constructs will be defined and discussed in the following five chapters.

CHAPTER 2

Cultural Desire

*"The best and most beautiful things in the
world cannot be seen or even touched.
They must be felt with the heart."*
Helen Keller

Cultural desire is the spiritual and pivotal construct of cultural competence that provides the energy source and foundation for one's journey towards cultural competence. **Cultural desire is defined as the motivation of the healthcare professional to "want to" engage in the process of becoming culturally competent; not the "have to"** (Campinha-Bacote, 1998). This motivation is genuine and authentic, with no hidden agendas. Rogers (1951) states that genuineness, or congruence, is the very basic ability of a person to read his own inner experiencing and allow the quality of this inner experiencing to be apparent in the relationship.

Caring and Love

The concepts of caring and love are central to the construct of cultural desire. Cultural desire is based on the humanistic value of caring and the spiritual aspect of loving one another (Campinha-Bacote, 2003b). We are all unique individuals who belong to the same race – the human race, with similar basic human needs. Culturally responsive interventions are based on the premise that we recognize differences, but also build upon similarities. Our goal in providing culturally responsive health care is to find this common ground.

May (1975) describes care as "a state in which something does matter; it is the source of human tenderness." It has been said that people do not care how much you know, until they first know how much you care. This type of caring "comes from the heart; not from the mouth" (Campinha-Bacote, 1998). The goal is not to offer comments that are politically correct (words from the mouth), but rather to offer comments to the client that reflect true caring (words from the heart).

Van Hooft (1999) asserts that caring is a virtue and applied to the health professions, the virtue of caring should be seen as a practical comportment towards others, which has the goal of enhancing the health-related existence of others (p. 193). Van Hooft further suggests that the motivation of caring is importantly "other-directed" as opposed to self.

Chapman (2005) has a synergistic view of the concepts of love and caring, which he refers to as "radical loving care – creating a continuous chain of caring light around each patient" (p. 4). Chapman maintains, "Nurses don't choose the nursing profession to become rich. The best nurses choose caregiving out of a passion to serve" (p. 12). Cultural desire mandates a genuine passion and commitment to caring. Chapman (2005) maintains that individuals who are primarily committed to serving others above themselves are characterized by having a "Servant's Heart" (p. 66). A Servant's Heart symbolizes love's greatest expression, which assumes the full involvement of our best thought processes (Chapman, p. 10).

Sacrifice

Charles Dubois said, "The important thing is this: To be able at any moment to sacrifice what we are for what we could become." Cultural desire encompasses the capacity to sacrifice. One must be willing to sacrifice one's prejudice and biases towards culturally different clients in order to develop cultural desire. Howard (2003) adds that we must also sacrifice our "proprietary assumptions of our own rightness and our unreflective grip on our own certainty." This type of sacrifice involves the moral commitment to care for all clients, regardless of their cultural values, beliefs or practices. However, this task may be difficult when caring for challenging clients who engage in behaviors that may be in direct moral conflict with the healthcare professional (e.g., abortion, spousal abuse, sexual addictions).

For example, how does a healthcare professional care for an Arab client whose political and/or religious beliefs are in direct contrast to their beliefs? As healthcare professionals we do not have to accept the client's belief system, however, we must treat each person as a unique human being worthy and deserving of our love and care. In this sense, cultural desire is expressed in terms of human dignity, human rights, social justice and equity (Campinha-Bacote, 2006).

Social Justice

Cultural competence must be based on a commitment to social justice. Culturally competent individuals have the skills necessary to break down systems of practice that perpetuate inequities (Ndura, n.d.). Martin Luther King Jr. once said, "Of all forms of inequality, injustice in health care is the most shocking and inhumane" (King, n.d.) Stacks et al. (2004) calls for "socially just culturally competence" and asserts that true cultural competence necessitates an understanding of social inequalities and how they affect individuals and communities.

Research continues to demonstrate a direct correlation between inequality and negative health outcomes and it is because of this link that healthcare professionals must consciously connect cultural competence with social justice. Stacks et. al (2004) contends that when cultural competence partners with social justice, we can finally achieve equality in health outcomes for all, regardless of race/ethnicity, language, gender, religion, or sexual orientation.

Several professional healthcare organizations have demonstrated a commitment to social justice. *The American Nurses Association's Position Statement on Ethics and Human Rights* (1991) supports this view, as evidenced in their following statements:

- Human beings deserve respect as ends in themselves, and therefore, deserve health care services that are equitable in terms of accessibility, availability, affordability and quality;
- Justice requires that the differences among persons and groups are to be valued. When those differences contribute to the unequal distribution of the quality and quantity of health care, then remedial actions are obligated;
- Because nursing care is an essential but sometimes limited commodity, allocation of care is a pressing issue that cannot be effectively addressed when specific individuals are excluded or when the burdens of limited access are borne by particular groups;
- The principle of justice applies to nurses as providers as well as to nurses as recipients of care. ANA is committed to addressing the need for racial and ethnic diversity among nurses. Such diversity is a critical element in providing fair and equitable care.

The Transcultural Nursing Society (TCNS) has made a recommitment "to safeguard human rights and quality health care through the discovery and implementation of culturally competent care" by recently developing a *Position Statement on Human Rights* (Andrews et al., 2007). This document serves as evidence that they are "committed to the rights of all peoples to enjoy their full human potential, including the highest attainable standard of health."

The culturally competent person must become aware and sensitized to the overt and covert social inequities faced by others. This requires a community perception of the challenges of social justice for all. Therefore, a major step toward socially just cultural competence is to enter into community partnerships. "The process of becoming culturally competent now moves outward from the individual, into the community" (Stacks et al., 2004, p. 5).

Humility

Humility or humbleness is a quality of seeing the greatness in others and coming into the realization of the dignity and worth of others. Healthcare professionals who are humble have a genuine desire to discover how their patients think and feel differently from them. A humble person is generally thought to be someone who does not think that he or she is better or more important than others. However, humility does not command us to consider ourselves lower in stature. Humility is not thinking less of yourself; but thinking of yourself, less.

In integrating humility into the construct of cultural desire, it is helpful to view it as the virtue of serving others. Matthew 20:26-27 states, "…but whoever wishes to become great among you shall be your servant, and whoever wishes to be first among you shall be your slave" (*New American Standard Bible*, 2002). The virtue of humility, in this sense, is directed toward serving our fellow man.

However, there is said to be a paradox in possessing humility, for when we become aware of our humility and openly acknowledge it, we've lost it. This begs the question: "Is it possible to seek or learn humility? Drawing from the field of theology, Ells (n.d.) argues that there are theological ways to humble oneself that are found in the books of Proverbs, Philippians, Corinthians, Matthew, Thessalonians, Ephesians and James (*New American Standard Bible*, 2002). His examples include accepting a lowly place, receiving correction and feedback from others graciously, choosing to serve others, being quick to forgive, cultivating a grateful heart, purposely speaking well of others, and acknowledging your wrongdoings to others.

Tervalon and Murray-Garcia (1998) have applied the concept of humility to the process of becoming culturally competent healthcare professionals and coined the term, "cultural humility." Cultural humility is defined as a life-long commitment to self-evaluation and self-critique, re-addressing the power imbalances in the patient-healthcare professional relationship and developing mutually beneficial partnerships with communities on behalf of individuals and defined populations.

Summary

Cultural desire comes from one's aspiration, and not out of one's desperation (Campinha-Bacote, 2005a). Cultural desire includes a genuine passion and commitment to be open and flexible with others; a respect for differences, yet a commitment to build upon similarities; a willingness to learn from clients and others as cultural informants; and a sense of humility (Campinha-Bacote, 2003b). As eloquently stated by Napoleon Hill, "The starting point of all achievement is desire," however, he adds, "Weak desires bring weak results." It is desire that creates our future and if healthcare professionals want to create a future of rendering culturally responsive services, it will have to be driven by desire. Desire is the fuel necessary to draw us into a personal journey towards cultural competence (Campinha-Bacote, 2003c).

CHAPTER 3

Cultural Awareness

"To learn about other people is science,
to learn to know yourself is intelligence."
Chinese Proverb

Cultural awareness is the deliberate self-examination and in-depth exploration of our personal biases, stereotypes, prejudices and assumptions that we hold about individuals who are different from us. It is an affective or attitudinal construct, which involves "insight into personal cultural heritage, the disciplinary heritage into which one has been socialized as a health care provider, and the organizational culture within which services are delivered . . ." (Schim et al., 2007, p. 107). However, personal biases are so ingrained in one's mind that they are not always directly available to our conscious thinking.

Van Ryn and Burke (2000) examined the biases of 193 physician-patient interactions with 842 patients (57% white and 43% black) in regard to the degree in which the patient's race and socio-economic status affected physicians' perceptions of patients during the encounter. This study revealed that physicians rated African American patients as less intelligent, less educated, more likely to abuse drugs and alcohol, more likely not to comply with medical advice, and more likely to lack social support than white patients, even after factors such as the patients' income and education were taken into consideration.

The most serious barrier to culturally competent care is not a lack of knowledge of the details of any given cultural orientation, but the providers' failure to develop self-awareness and a respectful attitude toward diverse points of view (Hunt, 2001). Cullnan

(1999) adds, "I believe we must live an 'examined life': acting consciously to examine

how we think about, how we hear, and how we act toward others." Without becoming

aware of the impact our cultural values have on our interaction with others, there is risk

that the healthcare professional may engage in cultural imposition. Cultural imposition is

the tendency to impose ones beliefs, values and patterns of behavior upon another culture

(Leininger, 1978).

In seeking cultural awareness there must be a commitment to cultural openness –

"a lifelong stance that promotes cultural self awareness and continuing development of

transcultural skills" (Wenger, 1998, p. 64). Wenger further adds that cultural openness

connotes both cognition and emotion, whereby the human will is engaged in learning

about transcultural similarities and differences. Lara (1997) suggests the following self-

examination and self-awareness questions to consider when answering the question,

"Where are you in your journey toward cultural awareness?"

1. What cultural/ethnic group, socio-economic class, religion, age, and community do you belong to?
2. What experiences have you had with people from cultural groups, socio-economic classes, religions, age groups, or communities different from yourself?
3. How did you feel about them?
4. When you were growing up, what did your parents and significant others say about people who were different from your family?
5. What about your cultural/ethnic group, religion, socio-economic class, age or community did you feel embarrassing or wish you could change?
6. What personal qualities do you have that will help you establish interpersonal relations with persons from other cultures?
7. What personal qualities may be detrimental?

Cultural Consciousness Continuum

To better understand the dynamics of cultural awareness, it may be useful to imagine cultural awareness along a continuum that ranges from unconscious incompetence to unconscious competence (Campinha-Bacote, 1996; Purnell, 1998). There are four levels of cultural competence: *unconscious incompetence, conscious incompetence, conscious competence* and *unconscious competence.* These four stages are directly related to one's level of cultural awareness or consciousness regarding interactions with individuals outside one's cultural group.

Unconscious incompetence is being unaware that one is lacking cultural knowledge. The healthcare professional is not aware that cultural differences exist between themselves and the client. One expert describes this as the "cultural blind spot syndrome" (Buchwald et al., 1994). Specifically, the healthcare professional may assume that there are no cultural differences because a particular client may look and behave much the same way the healthcare professional does. One example of the cultural blind spot syndrome is when the healthcare professional may believe that because a client is of the same ethnic group, they share similar values, beliefs, lifestyles and practices. This may be a faulty assumption based on the concept of intra-cultural variation. Intra-cultural variation means that there is as much variation within cultural groups as across cultural groups.

Conscious incompetence is being aware that one is lacking knowledge about another cultural group (Purnell, 1998). Here, the healthcare professional is keenly aware that cultural differences exist. The healthcare professional may have realized this by attending a workshop on cultural diversity, reading an article or book on the topic, discussing cultural issues with peers, or having a direct cross-cultural experience with a client from a different cultural background. These healthcare professionals possess the "know that" knowledge, but not the "know how" knowledge. They know that culture plays a key role when interacting with others, but they do not know how to effectively communicate with clients from different cultural backgrounds.

Conscious competence is described by Purnell (1998) as the conscious act of learning about the client's culture, verifying generalizations and providing culturally relevant interventions. The consciously competent healthcare professional has personally experienced cross-cultural interactions and is extremely aware that cultural differences must be respected and understood in order to have successful and effective cross-cultural interactions. These healthcare professionals are deliberate in applying the cultural knowledge and principles they have learned, however, because of their limited encounters with clients from different cultural groups, these healthcare professionals may not feel comfortable when interacting with culturally diverse clients. One possible reason for this discomfort is the fear of not being "politically correct." Healthcare professionals at this level are overly conscious of doing and saying the right thing. At times, their political correctness can actually interfere with effective communication.

Unconscious competence is the ability of the healthcare professional to spontaneously provide culturally responsive care to clients from a diverse culture. These healthcare professionals have experienced many encounters with culturally diverse clients and have developed an intuitive grasp of how to easily and effectively communicate in cross-cultural encounters. The timing of unconsciously competent healthcare professionals is always accurate and they appear to be "a natural" when observed interacting with clients from culturally diverse backgrounds. However, Purnell (1998) states that "unconscious competence is difficult to accomplish ... most healthcare providers can expect to reach only the conscious competence stage of cultural development" (p. 2).

Interacting Styles

In progressing through the stages of cultural awareness, there are different interaction styles that the healthcare professional may consciously or unconsciously operate in. Although Bell and Evans (1981) identified five basic interpersonal styles in terms of how non-black counselors might interact with a black client, these interacting styles can be applied to healthcare professionals interacting with clients from ethnically and racially diverse culture groups. These interacting styles are *overt racism and hostility, covert (hidden) racism, cultural ignorance, color blind,* and *culturally liberated.*

Overt racism is when the healthcare professional interacts out of deep-seated prejudices that he/she has toward a particular cultural group. The healthcare professional will use the power of his/her attitudes and behaviors to dehumanize the client. This interaction is very unlikely to produce any positive outcomes (Bell & Evans, 1981).

Covert racism is an interacting style in which the healthcare professional is aware of his/her fears of a specific cultural group, but knows that open expression of those attitudes is inappropriate. The healthcare professional attempts to hide or "cover-up" the true feelings beneath the surface of the healthcare professional façade (Bell & Evans, 1981, p.15). Bell and Evans add that, more often than not, this interaction will betray the healthcare professional's true feelings and lack of empathy for the client (p. 15).

Cultural ignorance is an interacting style in which the healthcare professional has had little or no prior exposure to the specific cultural group. This healthcare professional may experience fear due to his/her inability to relate to the client. Bell and Evans (1981) state that this fear of failure becomes a self-fulfilling prophecy.

The *color blind* healthcare professional has made a conscious decision that he/she is committed to equality for all people and therefore treats all people alike, regardless of cultural background. This healthcare professional denies the reality of cultural differences that are important for effective interactions.

Finally, the *culturally liberated* healthcare professional does not fear cultural differences and is aware of his/her attitude towards specific cultural groups. This healthcare professional encourages the client to express feelings about their cultural and ethnic background and uses these feelings as a shared learning experience. Healthcare professionals must be aware of what interacting style they are operating in and strive toward a culturally liberated interacting style.

Lethal "Isms"

Wonders (2006) asserts that ". . . the root of all 'isms' is an insatiable addiction to power or its attributes, specifically what is described as 'power-over,' as differentiated from 'power-to.'" In examining one's biases, healthcare professionals must be cognitive of the many lethal "isms" that continue to afflict healthcare delivery. Ageism, sexism, ethnocentrism, classism, ableism, and racism are just a few examples of isms that can negatively affect the healthcare professional-patient relationship and health outcomes. *The American Nurses Association's Position Statement on Discrimination and Racism in Health Care* (2002), states that, "Discrimination and racism continue to be a part of the fabric and tradition of American society and have adversely affected minority

populations, the health care system in general, and the profession of nursing."

Beer (1998) states that "we can challenge and control our prejudices and biases to

some extent...however, what we can't easily change is the system we are part of, the fact

that our positional identity gives us a relative advantage or disadvantage whether we seek

to have it or not. Therefore, in seeking cultural awareness, we need to scrutinize our

position in society and our experiences of privilege and oppression and ask the question,

"How have these experiences shaped our worldview?"

In examining the position of privilege, both McIntosh (1988) and Cullnan (1999)

describe the concept of unearned privileges of the dominant culture in the United States.

McIntosh (1988) refers to the unearned privilege of the dominant culture as *white*

privilege. She states, "as a white person I was taught to see racism only in individual acts

of meanness, not in invisible systems conferring dominance on my group." McIntosh

acknowledges that being white (white privilege) allows her an invisible package of

unearned assets that she can count on cashing in each day. Some examples she gives of

white privilege are:

- I can go shopping alone most of the time, pretty well assured that I will
  not be followed or harassed.
- I can be sure that my children will be given curricula materials that
  testify to the existence of their race.
- I can be sure that if I ask to talk to "the person in charge" I will be
  facing a person of my race.
- I can be sure if I need legal or medical help my race will not act
  against me.

Cullnan (1999) describes the unearned privileges of the dominant culture as the

"*three principle presumptions of dominant culture privilege.*" The first presumption is

the presumption of innocence. Cullnan, being of the dominant culture, remarks, "When

33

something goes wrong around me, people do not look to me first, or even second, as a probable cause of the problem." From this perspective, those not privileged in the dominant culture are frequently seen as guilty until proven innocent. The second presumption is *the presumption of worthiness* - "the presumption that I am worthy, deserving and good enough to receive attention, services, respect, and the benefit of the doubt" (Cullnan). This phenomenon is clearly evident in medical care, in which a large body of research supports the findings that racial and ethnic minorities in the United States receive lower quality health care than whites, even when insurance status, income, age and severity of condition are comparable (Smedley et al., 2002). The last presumption is *the presumption of competence.* This presumption assumes that the dominant culture is competent, while assuming incompetence of cultural groups such as ethnic minority groups, women and people with disabilities. We have seen discrimination based on disability necessitating congress to pass the Americans with Disabilities Act. This legislation was an attempt to correct the stereotypical connection between disabilities and incompetence (Cullnan). At times, African Americans have been described in the media as being " very articulate" and "bright," a comment noticeably assuming that most African Americans are not articulate or smart.

Cullnan (1999) gives the following rules to address dominant culture privilege:

1. Tolerate no one. By merely tolerating anyone, I am treating them as less than human being, fully worthy of my attention.
2. In the absence of direct evidence to the contrary, give everyone the presumption of innocence, the presumption of worthiness and the presumption of competence.
3. Keeping my own humility alive. It is easy to forget that I do not live on the "front lines." I can choose when and how long to go there.
4. Refuse to characterize the lived experiences of others as "isolated incidents. Challenge this characterization when I hear it from others.

5. Listen especially hard when it is difficult to listen. When I notice myself getting defensive as hearing from people of non-dominant groups that what I. . . was offensive, I try to remember to take a deep breath and listen carefully…
6. Take the opportunity to use my position of privilege (having the presumptions of innocence, worthiness and competence) to make sure that others, who may not have privilege, have their voices heard.

Summary

Beer (1998) states, "all of us carry stereotypes and prejudices--it is in the air we breathe." Unfortunately, healthcare professionals often reflect the attitudes and discriminatory practices of their society. A healthcare professional's cultural and ethnic background can affect interpreting, assigning meaning to, and creating value judgments about their patients. In addition, the lack of awareness of one's biases can result in the lack of diagnostic clarity. The process of gaining cultural awareness is an important first step in one's journey towards recognizing personal biases, prejudice, and discriminatory practices. Pedersen (1988) suggests the following techniques to stimulate cultural awareness: (1) experiential exercises (role plays, role reversals, simulations); (2) field trips; (3) guided self-study with a reading list; (4) critical incidents; (5) panel discussions; (6) audio-visual presentations; (7) interviews with consultants and experts; and (8) bicultural observations. Pedersen's goal in this awareness focus is to assist the healthcare professional to become aware of the contrast and conflict between their background and that of the client's cultural background. However, solely becoming aware of isms and one's biases towards other cultures does not insure the rendering of culturally competent care. The healthcare professional's journey towards cultural competence must move beyond cultural awareness and include insight into other components of cultural competence.

CHAPTER 4

Cultural Knowledge

"We shall not cease from explorations;
and the end of all our exploring
will be to arrive where we started. . .
and know the place for the first time."
T.S. Eliot

Cultural knowledge is the process of seeking and obtaining a sound educational base about culturally diverse groups (Campinha-Bacote, 1998). Healthcare professionals can obtain this knowledge from several sources: 1) academic textbooks on the topic of transcultural healthcare and related topics (Jeffreys, 2006); 2) computer-based programs such as interactive e-learning modules designed to improve one's ability to deliver quality care to culturally diverse patient populations (United States Department of Health and Human Services Office of Minority Health's *Culturally Competent Nursing Modules,* 2007); 3) video programs (*Quality Care for Diverse Populations Video,* 2007); 4) novels, such as *The Spirit Catches You and You Fall Down* (Fadiman, 1997); and 5) spiritual sources, such as the Bible (Campinha-Bacote, 2005b). In acquiring this knowledge, healthcare professionals must focus on the integration of three specific issues: health-related beliefs practices and cultural values; disease incidence and prevalence; and treatment efficacy (Lavizzo-Mourey, 1996).

Health-Related Beliefs

Obtaining knowledge regarding the client's health-related beliefs, practices and values necessitates an understanding of their worldview. One of the most influential factors for understanding an individual's behavior is to understand their worldview. An individual's worldview becomes the foundation for all actions and interpretations. Nichols' (1987) theoretical model, The Philosophical Aspects of Cultural Differences, asserts that a cultural groups' worldview includes *axiology, epistemology, logic* and *process. Axiology* is what a culture values the highest. Nichols contends that for some African Americans, the highest value lies in interpersonal relationships between persons. In contrast, some European Americans' highest value lies in the acquisition of objects or what we would refer to as materialism. *Epistemology* refers to how a cultural group comes to know truth or knowledge. For example, some African Americans come to knowledge affectively, or through feelings. *Logic* refers to a cultural group's nature of reasoning, while *process* refers to a cultural group's view of the nature of relationships in the world. There are several websites that provide healthcare professionals with the values, beliefs, lifeways and practices of cultural groups (Appendix B).

Disease Incidence and Prevalence

Disease incidence and prevalence is the second issue healthcare professionals must address when obtaining cultural knowledge. Disease incidence varies among ethnic groups and healthcare professionals that do not have accurate epidemiological data to guide decisions about treatment, health education, screening, and treatment programs may have a negative impact on healthcare outcomes. Common diseases and health conditions found among ethnic groups are reflected in the following list:

Chinese Americans
Hepatitis B
Tuberculosis
Diabetes mellitus
Pancreatic cancer in women

Arab Americans
　　Sickle cell anemia
　　Thalassemias
　　Familial hypercholesterolemia
　　Mediterranean fever

Jewish Americans
　　Genetic disorders (e.g., Tay-Sachs disease, Gaucher's disease,
　　　Niemann-Pick disease, Bloom's syndrome, and Riely-Day
　　　Syndrome)
　　Inflammatory bowel disease
　　Karposi's sarcoma in men of Ashkenazi descent

Mexican Americans
　　Cancer
　　Alcoholism and drug abuse
　　Diabetes Mellitus
　　Dental diseases

Navajo Indians
　　Severe combined immunodeficiency syndrome, unrelated to AIDS
　　Genetically prone blindness
　　Diabetes Mellitus
　　Navajo neuropathy
　　Albinism

In addition to these diseases and health conditions found among ethnic groups,

some examples of health disparities prevalent among the African American population

are:

1. Compared with hypertension in other ethnic groups, hypertension among African Americans is more severe, more resistant to treatment, begins at a younger age, and the consequence is significantly worst target organ damage (Brewster, et al., 2004; Moore, 2005, p. 23).
2. African American women face greater disparities in incidence of infant mortality and morbidity. They have higher rates of delivering premature/low birth infants and the rate of death due to prematurity/low birth weight for black infants is almost four times that for whites.
3. The incidence of type 2 diabetes in African Americans is among the highest in the world (Sowers et al., 2002). African Americans experience double the prevalence of complications related to their diabetes.
4. African Americans experience higher overall cancer incidence and mortality rates and lower five-year survival rates when compared to non-Hispanic white, Native American, Hispanic, Alaskan Native, Asian American, and Pacific Islander population groups (Underwood & Powell, 2006).

5. African Americans have a disproportionally higher rate of poor asthma outcomes, including hospitalizations and deaths. Deaths due to asthma are three times more common among African Americans than among whites (The Asthma and Allergy Foundation of America and the National Pharmaceutical Council, 2006).
6. In 2003, African Americans, who make up approximately 12% of the US population, accounted for half of the HIV/AIDS cases diagnosed.

Treatment Efficacy

Treatment efficacy is the third issue to address in the process of obtaining cultural knowledge. This involves obtaining knowledge in such areas as ethnic pharmacology. Ethnic pharmacology has also been referred to as cross-cultural pharmacology, transcultural pharmacology, ethno pharmacology, and interethnic pharmacology (Pi & Simpson, 2005; Edmond, 1998; Burroughs et al., 2003; Munoz & Hilgenberg, 2005). Ethnic pharmacology can be defined as the field of study that investigates the impact that culture, environment, genetics, bio-physiology and psychosocial factors have on the prescribing and metabolism of, and response to therapeutic medications.

Ethnic pharmacology has sparked much controversy, for many take the position that racial categories are more a societal construct than a scientific one and argue that caution must be exercised in promoting drugs for specific ethnic groups (Ferdinand, 2006). Others add that ethnic pharmacology is a form of racial profiling and could easily lead to stereotyping and discrimination (Schwartz, 2001). In contrast, Satel (2000) maintains that although race is a rough biological classification, healthcare professionals must not be blind to its clinical application and the sound research that has been conducted in this area. Considering these divergent viewpoints, it is recommended to use caution when obtaining and applying knowledge in the field of ethnic pharmacology. Healthcare professionals must be aware of possible clinical applications of this field of study, while at the same time demonstrating a respect for individual differences and similarities across racial groups.

There are many factors involved in determining responses to a specific drug among ethnic groups. These factors include *environmental* concerns, the *cultural beliefs and practices* of both client and healthcare professional, *genetics*, and *generic drug substitution.*

An *environmental factor* noted among ethnic groups is diet. Diet has been routinely disregarded in the standard pharmacology textbooks, except for when diet has obvious effects on dosing. However, certain fruits and vegetables affect the C4P 1A2 isoenzyme that metabolizes haloperidol and clozapine. For example, a glass of grapefruit juice inhibits C4P 1A2,5 whereas broccoli, Brussels sprouts, and cabbage induce that isoenzyme. Psychotherapeutic medications, such as antidepressants, that require fat in order to be absorbed are not as effective in patients with exceptionally low body fat or differing fat metabolism (Wandler, 2003). This is a factor to consider when caring for Ghanaians, who may differ in fat metabolism as compared to Americans (Banini et al., 2003).

Malnutrition can also influence drug response. Protein, vitamin, and mineral deficiencies can hamper the function of metabolic enzymes, and alter the body's ability to absorb or eliminate a psychotherapeutic drug. This may pose a problem for newly arriving refugees from Ethiopia/Eritrea and other East African countries where malnutrition is considered a major medical problem. When there are unexplained variations in a patient's response to a medication, it is imperative for the healthcare professional to assess the patient's dietary habits.

An example of a *cultural* factor that can influence drug response in ethnic groups is the client's use of herbs. Ethnopharmacology, also called phytomedicine, is the study of herbs and their medicinal properties. Many cultural and ethnic groups use herbs to treat illnesses and maintain health, which may interfere with the prescribed medication. Marin and Escobar (2001) report that Hispanics use herbal remedies more often than non-Hispanics. Eisenberg et al. (1998) conducted a large-scale study in which they found 15 million adults were at risk for drug-herb interaction. Other studies reveal that approximately 40% of clients enrolled in health maintenance organizations (HMOs) were on herbs without their primary care provider's knowledge (Eisenberg et al., 1993).

Another *cultural* factor that can affect drug response among ethnic groups is the healthcare professional's biases and prejudices toward culturally diverse groups. This prejudice can lead to misdiagnosis and over-medication. DelBello et al., (1999) found in a study with adolescents that although there were no differences in psychotic symptoms among African Americans and Caucasians, African American adolescents still received more antipsychotic medications. There are several possible explanations for this discrepancy; however, DelBello cites that one possibility is that clinicians perceived African Americans to be more aggressive and more psychotic and thus prescribed the antipsychotic.

Genetics also plays a role in drug response among ethnic groups. The cytochrome P450 system contains over 200 genetically determined enzymes known to regulate drug metabolism. Certain types of genetic variations (allele frequencies) of importance in the metabolism of drugs are more common in some ethnic groups than others. For example, half of the Chinese and Japanese populations have a polymorphism of the gene encoding

42

the enzyme alcohol dehydrogenase 2, resulting in an inactive variant of that enzyme that has been associated with Asian alcohol hypersensitivity and the risk for esophageal cancer (Takeshita, 2000). Caucasian or African populations rarely show this isozyme variation. Therapeutic ranges of lithium can also differ among ethnic groups. Lin et al. (1986) reported that the therapeutic range of lithium for manic patients in Japan and Taiwan to be 0.4 - 0.8 mEq/L, as compared to 0.6 - 1.2 mEq/L for patients in the United States. In another research study, Schaeffeler et al. (2001) found that a genetic mutation may make certain antiretroviral treatments less effective in Africans and African Americans.

Generic substitution of a trade drug can be an issue for certain ethnic groups. While 10% of the active drug component of a generic drug can differ, there is a greater range allowed in the filler. These fillers may pose a problem for specific ethnic groups. For instance, lactose, a common filler constituent, may be relied on to a greater degree by pharmaceutical companies; however, they may cause unpleasant side effects in susceptible ethnic populations (Levy, 1993). Certain insurance company's prescribing formulary may not take this factor into account and assume that there is no difference in drug response when taking a generic verses a trade name drug.

Diagnostic Clarity

In addition to treatment efficacy, cultural knowledge is needed in the area of diagnostic clarity among cultural groups. Diagnostic clarity includes the role of the healthcare professional and their ability to maintain diagnostic objectivity in cross-cultural situations. The Surgeon General's Report on Mental Health states that persons from racial and ethnic groups are often misdiagnosed within mental health systems (U.S.

43

Department of Health and Human Services, 2001). Therefore, diagnostic clarity becomes an important factor to consider when providing psychiatric and mental health care to racial and ethnic groups, for it can be confounded by differences in behavioral expressions among various cultural groups.

The select expression of an illness by a culture is referred to as a culture-bound illness or syndrome. Knowledge of culture-bound illnesses is necessary to maintain diagnostic clarity and prevent potential misdiagnosis among cultural groups. Leff (1981) defines culture-bound syndromes as features of an illness that vary from culture to culture. Susto (fright) and mal ojo (evil eye) are two culture-bound syndromes noted in some Hispanic/Latino populations. *Susto,* or soul loss, is the belief that a frightening experience can cause illness. When this fright occurs, it is believed that the soul of the victim has been captured by spirits. Symptoms include anorexia, listlessness, apathy and withdrawal. If not aware of this culture-bound illness, healthcare professionals may misdiagnose susto as clinical depression. This misdiagnosis can further lead to inappropriate treatment. *Mal ojo* embodies the belief that social relations contain dangers to an individual. It is stated that women and children are more susceptible to this illness because they are weaker. The belief is that a strong person with "vista Fuerte" (strong vision) can exert a negative power over the weaker person causing them to become ill. Symptoms such as fevers, rashes, nervousness and irritability can appear abruptly in cases of mal ojo.

Since mal ojo and susto, as well as other culture-bound illnesses, can closely mimic psychopathology, there is a serious concern for misdiagnosis among cultural groups. In response to the concern of misdiagnosis of ethnic groups and the need for diagnostic clarity, the *Diagnostic Statistical Manual of Mental Disorders-IV* (*DSM-IV*) proposed an outline (Cultural Formulation) for a systematic evaluation of the impact of the client's cultural context (American Psychiatric Association, 1994). This outline includes assessment of the cultural identity of the client, cultural explanations of the client's illness, cultural elements of the relationship between the client and the mental health professional, cultural factors related to the psychosocial environment and levels of functioning, and the overall cultural assessment for diagnostic care. The *DSM-IV* hoped to address the issue of clinician bias by developing this Cultural Formulation, however, Neighbors (2003) claims that the problem is that there have been no systematic assessments of the usefulness of the Cultural Formulation, and as a result we need to explore its value in the diagnostic process.

The *DSM-IV* also provides health professionals with a glossary list of best-studied cultural-bound syndromes and idioms of distress that one may encounter during a cross-cultural assessment. This resource can be extremely helpful to clinicians, however, Marsella (2003) asserts,

> "It is notable that the DSM-IV provides a list of culture-bound disorders and it does note that these should be considered. But, it stops short of providing specific diagnostic procedures for assessing culture-bound disorders and for warning diagnosticians of the risks of using DSM-IV categories for non-Western patients" (p. 16).

Marsella furthers adds that if culture-bound syndromes are limited to specific cultures, who defines what are the criteria for mental illness - American or European psychiatrists?

Interacting Styles Within Cultural Groups

In obtaining cultural knowledge it is also important to understand the different interacting styles found within cultural groups. Bell and Evans (1981) assert that there are four distinctive interacting styles; *acculturated, culturally-immersed, traditional,* and *bicultural.* The *acculturated* interpersonal style is when a client from a culturally diverse group makes a conscious or unconscious decision to reject the values, beliefs, practices and general behaviors associated with his/her own cultural group. In contrast, the *culturally-immersed* client rejects all values, except those held by their cultural group. These clients are often labeled as militant or difficult. This client becomes immersed in his/her culture as a survival mechanism. The *traditional* interpersonal style is noted when the client neither rejects nor accepts their cultural identity. They do not disclose information about their cultural practices. Finally, the *bicultural* interacting style demonstrates the pride that a client has for their history and cultural traditions, while still feeling connected and comfortable in the mainstream world. These clients live in both worlds- but at an emotional expense.

Culturally diverse clients who choose to operate under a bicultural interacting style take on the risk of being negatively labeled by their own cultural group as "trying to act white." African Americans operating in a bicultural interacting style are referred to as "Oreos" - black on the outside, but white on the inside; while Native Americans are called "Apples" - red on the outside, but white on the inside. Similarly, Hispanics/ Latinos are labeled as "Coconuts" by their own cultural group - brown on the outside, but white on the inside and Asians are referred to as "Bananas" - yellow on the outside, but white on the inside.

It is important to understand Bell and Evans' (1981) interacting styles of culturally diverse groups when rendering care, for an acculturated client may be offended by your offer of culturally relevant services, while the culturally-immersed client will demand these services.

Summary

In obtaining cultural knowledge, it is critical to remember the concept of intra-cultural variation – there are marked differences within cultural groups. For example, Hispanics/Latinos are not a homogenous group, but rather reflect a very heterogeneous group comprised of such subgroups as Puerto Ricans, Mexicans, Cubans, and Peruvians. No individual is a stereotype of one's culture of origin, but rather a unique blend of the diversity found within each culture, a unique accumulation of life experiences, and the process of acculturation to other cultures.

It is important to keep in mind that cultures are constantly evolving and no healthcare professional can hope to be completely familiar with the health beliefs and practices of all their clients, nor can clients realistically expect such encyclopedia awareness from the healthcare professional (Recommendations from the Minnesota Public Health Associations Immigrant Health Task Force, 1996). In addition, healthcare professionals cannot solely rely on textbooks and websites for cultural knowledge; they must also develop the ability necessary to obtain cultural knowledge directly from the client. Therefore, the healthcare professional must develop the skill to conduct a cultural assessment with each client.

CHAPTER 5

Cultural Skill

"With the gift of listening
comes the gift of healing."
Catherine De Hueck Doherty

Cultural skill is the ability to collect relevant cultural data regarding the client's presenting problem, as well as accurately performing a culturally based, physical assessment in a culturally sensitive manner (Campinha-Bacote, 2003a). This process involves learning the skills of how to conduct a cultural assessment and perform culturally based physical assessments. The goal of a cultural assessment is to obtain accurate information from the client that will allow the healthcare professional to diagnose the client's presenting problem and formulate a mutually acceptable and culturally relevant treatment plan. Leininger (1978) defines a cultural assessment as a "systematic appraisal or examination of individuals, groups, and communities as to their cultural beliefs, values and practices to determine explicit needs and intervention practices within the context of the people being served" (pp. 85-86).

Cultural Assessment Tools

The literature is saturated with cultural assessment tools, frameworks and mnemonics that can assist healthcare professionals in conducting a cultural assessment. A review of these tools is useful in providing healthcare professionals with a wide selection of cultural questions, mnemonics, domains and/or phenomena that can be integrated into their existing health history or assessment form. This framework (Integrated Model Approach to Conducting Cultural Assessments) consists of the following steps: (1) review several cultural assessment tools; (2) consider your discipline's and specialty's purpose in conducting an assessment; (3) consider your personal assets and liabilities as an interviewer; (4) integrate selected questions from specific cultural assessment tools that will augment your existing assessment form to yield culturally relevant data; and (5) establish your own personal style of incorporating cultural content into your patient assessment (Campinha-Bacote, 2003a). If a cultural assessment is conducted in this manner, culture is not singled-out, but rather appropriately incorporated into the client's overall assessment.

There are cultural assessment tools that describe domains or phenomena to be considered when assessing a client's cultural background (Leininger, 2002; Purnell, 2003; Giger & Davidhizar, 2003). Purnell (2003) developed an organizing framework consisting of 12 domains, which are common to all cultures:

1. Overview, inhabited localities and topography
2. Communication
3. Family roles and organization
4. Workforce issues
5. Biocultural ecology
6. High-risk health behaviors
7. Nutrition
8. Pregnancy and childbearing
9. Death rituals
10. Spirituality
11. Health-care practices
12. Health-care practitioners

Overview, inhabited localities and topography include the client's heritage and residence, reasons for migration and associated economic factors, educational status and occupation. The domain of *communication* involves knowing about the client's language and dialect, cultural communication patterns, temporal relationships and format for names. *Workforce issues* relate to the differences and conflicts that occur in the workplace setting. These issues include such factors as degree of assimilation and acculturation and issues related to professional autonomy. *Family roles and organization* require gaining information about family roles and priorities, alternative lifestyles and traditional families, and issues surrounding gender and head of household. *Biocultural ecology* is the specific domain that identifies the client's physical, biological and physiological variations. Examples of these variations are noted in drug metabolism and disease and health conditions. *High-risk health behaviors* include specific high-risk behaviors common among cultural groups. These behaviors may include the use of alcohol, tobacco and recreational drugs. The cultural domain, *nutrition*, includes the client's meaning of food, common food and food rituals, dietary practices for health promotion, and nutritional deficiencies and limitations. The domain, *pregnancy and childbearing practices*, includes obtaining knowledge about the client's culturally sanctioned and unsanctioned fertility practices; views toward pregnancy; and prescriptive, restrictive and taboo practices related to pregnancy, birthing and postpartum. *Death rituals* include how the client views death and euthanasia, rituals to prepare for death and bereavement, and burial practices. The domain of *spirituality* involves more than the client's religious affiliation. Spirituality encompasses religious practices, use of prayer, meaning of life and individual sources of strength, spiritual beliefs and healthcare practices related to these beliefs. *Health-care practices* include health-seeking behaviors and beliefs, responsibility for health-care, folklore practices, barriers to care, cultural responses to health and illness, beliefs regarding blood transfusions, organ donation and organ transplantation. The final domain of *health-care practitioner* includes the status, use and perceptions of traditional, magicoreligious practitioners, and biomedical healthcare professionals.

Giger and Davidhizar (2003) assert that their Transcultural Assessment Model provides healthcare professionals with a practical assessment tool for evaluating cultural variables that greatly minimizes the time needed to conduct a comprehensive assessment. These authors assert that culturally diverse care must take into account six cultural phenomena that vary with application and use, yet are evident in all cultural groups: (1) communication, (2) space, (3) social organization, (4) time, (5) environmental control, and (6) biological variation. The variable, *communication*, addresses both verbal and non-verbal communication, while the variable of *space* assesses issues regarding personal boundaries and interpersonal space. *Social organization* includes assessing such information as family structure and religious values, while the phenomenon of *time* refers to not only assessing how the client measures time, but their temporal perspective (past, present or future). *Environmental control* addresses the client's ability to plan activities that control nature. This variable includes the client' health practices. The final variable of *biological variations* includes the client's physical dimensions, enzymatic and genetic existence of diseases specific to their cultural group, and nutritional preferences and deficiencies.

Leininger (2002) encourages healthcare processionals to conduct a holistic "culturalological" assessment in the major areas of worldview and social structure factors which include cultural values, beliefs and practices; religious, philosophical or spiritual beliefs; economic factors; educational beliefs; technology views; kinship and social ties; and political and legal factors. Like Leininger, Kleinman (1980) is also interested in the clients' explanation of their illness. He refers to this as the client's Explanatory Model.

Explanatory models (EMs) are notions about sickness and its treatment. There are five

major questions that EMs seek to explain for illness episodes: (1) etiology, (2) time and

mode of onset of symptoms; (3) pathophysiology, (4) course of illness (including both

severity and type of sick role), and (5) treatment. Kleinman finds it useful to ask the

following open-ended questions in eliciting the details of the client's explanatory model:

1. What do you call your problem? What name does it have?
2. What do you think has caused your problem? Why do you think it started when it did?
3. What do you think your sickness does to you? How does it work?
5. How severe is it? Will it have a short or long course?
6. What do you fear the most about your sickness?
7. What are the chief problems your sickness has caused for you?
8. What kind of treatment do you think you should receive? What are the most important results you hope to receive from this treatment? (p. 106).

Due to the rapidly changing demographics of our growing multicultural world,

healthcare professionals will also encounter clients who may have recently migrated to

the United States, are refugees or who represent a second or third generation ethnic

group. Existing cultural assessment tools may not be appropriate for these clients.

Jacobsen (1988) and Chong (2002) have developed cultural assessment tools that address

issues relevant to clients who may have recently migrated to the United States.

Jacobsen (1988) refers to clients who have recently migrated to the United States

or who are refugees as ethnoculturally translocated clients. He proposes a five-stage

assessment tool. In Stage I, the healthcare professional obtains information on the

client's ethnocultural heritage, such as the culture of origin for both maternal and paternal

lines of the client's family. Stage II requires the healthcare professional to assess the circumstances leading to the client's ethno-cultural translocation(s). Stages III and IV

assess the client's intellectual and emotional perception of the development of the

family's niche in society since translocation, as well as the client's view of their cultural

adjustment as an individual. The final stage addresses information regarding the

healthcare professional's ethno-cultural background and areas of overlap or differences.

Although Chong (2002) developed the **GREET** model for Latino patients, this

mnemonic model can be easily adapted when assessing ethnoculturally translocated

patients from all ethnic groups. The GREET acronym stands for *Generation, Reason for*

Immigrating to the United States, Extended or Nuclear Family, Ethic Behavior, and *Time*

Living in the United States. It is important to assess the patient's *generational status* to

determine if the patient is an immigrant, second, third, or fourth generation. However,

healthcare professionals must be careful not to assume that third, fourth and fifth

generation patients are more acculturated than their first or second generation

counterparts (Rios-Ells et al., 2005). When asking questions about *reasons for*

immigrating to the United States, healthcare professionals are to be sensitive to the fact

that some immigrants may feel threatened due to potential lack of documentation as a

United States citizen. Knowing if the client lives in close proximity to either the

extended family or nuclear family provides valuable information about their source of

social support. Assessing such *ethnic behaviors* as preferences concerning food, music,

holidays, and recreational activities provides insight into the patient's culture as well as

provides information on health behaviors. Finally, assessing the amount of *time living in*

the United States will provide the healthcare professional with the patient's degree of

acculturation. For example, immigrants who have not resided in the United States for an extended period may tend to hold on to their traditional cultural beliefs. While this does not hold true for all ethnic groups, usually it can be expected that the longer the client has resided in the host country's culture the more chance that they may adopt some aspects of the host culture (Rios-Ellis et al., 2005, p. 78).

Cultural skill also involves the process of learning how to conduct a culturally sensitive medication assessment. Many cultural groups maintain attitudes and health beliefs regarding the properties and effects of medication that may affect the effectiveness of, or adherence to a drug. Therefore, healthcare professionals must become skillful in assessing this valuable patient history data. Gaw (2001) and Kudzma (2001) provide healthcare professionals with culturally sensitive questions to ask while conducting a medication history.

Gaw (2001) recommends the culturally sensitive medication assessment tool called "Clinician's Inquiry Into the Meaning of Taking Psychotropic Medications." This assessment tool asks questions regarding feelings about taking psychotropic medication, the meaning of taking psychotropic medications, religious beliefs regarding the taking of psychotropic medication, the benefits and risks of taking psychotropic medications, the meaning of the color, size, or form of medication, and questions concerning potential fears of losing control if taking psychotropic medication.

(Kudzma, 2001) suggests the following questions in assessing the cultural aspects of disease incidence and medication use among culturally diverse groups:

1. Is the patient knowledgeable of specific genetic conditions in his family that have a higher incidence in specific ethnic groups (e.g., sickle cell disease, G6PD deficiency, lactose intolerance)?
2. What are the patient's views of traditional or Western medicine?
3. Does the patient use any homeopathic, herbal, or cultural remedies?
4. How is nutritional intake influenced by the patient's culture?

5. What foods are eaten, and what are the timing and sequence of meals?
6. Are any specific nutritional differences noted that might impact drug absorption or metabolism (fat intake, food supplements)?
7. Does the patient smoke? Use alcohol? Use other drugs?
8. What are the patient's expectations regarding the effectiveness of the prescribed medication?

The healthcare professional's approach to the medication assessment must be done in a culturally sensitive manner. Munoz and Hilgenberg (2005) emphasize that it is best to ask patients specific questions about possible adverse effects of drugs rather than asking broad questions or waiting for the patient to voice concerns. Within some Asian cultures, patients infrequently complain, and with these patients you may need to ask specific questions to elicit important information about efficacy and potential side effects. For example, when interviewing a Chinese American patient taking haloperidol you might ask, "Have you noticed any unusual, uncontrolled movements?" to determine the presence or absence of extrapyramidal effects (Munoz & Hilgenberg).

Mnemonic Cultural Assessment Tools

To provide ease in the skill of conducting a cultural assessment, several authors have developed mnemonic cultural assessment tools (Fong, 1985; Carillo et al., 1999; Berlin & Fowkes, 1982; Stuart & Lieberman, 1993; Levine et al., 2000; Dobbie et al., 2003; Kagawa-Singer & Kassim-Lakha, 2003; Like, 2004).

Fong (1985) advocates the mnemonic **CONFHER,** as a framework for assessing the client's cultural background. CONFHER represents the cultural components of

C ommunication
O rientation
N utrition
F amily relationships
H ealth beliefs
E ducation
R eligion

Communication involves obtaining information on the client's language and dialect preference as well as nonverbal social customs. *Orientation* refers to the client's cultural identity. Asking the client what cultural group they identify with, allows the client to choose their own cultural orientation, rather than being labeled by the healthcare professional. Orientation also refers to how closely the client adheres to the traditional habits and values of their cultural group. *Nutritional* information can be obtained by asking such questions as: "Are there ethnic foods that you prefer?"; "Are there foods that you are encouraged to eat when sick?"; "Are there foods to be avoided because of your cultural origin, health status, or illness?" *Family relationships* involve assessing how the client defines family and how decisions are made in the family. Questions that can help in eliciting the client's *health beliefs* are: "Do you rely on any self-care or traditional folk medicine practices?"; "How do you explain your illness?"; and "How do you feel about being in the hospital?" *Educational* information can be obtained by assessing such factors as whether or not the client prefers to learn information by receiving printed literature, listening or viewing audio visual learning tools, by using hands-on experiential learning that involves trial and error or by didactic methods. *Religious* data involves the assessment of the client's religious or spiritual preference, beliefs, sacred rites, restrictions, and person that will be involved in their care to provide spiritual and religious comfort.

Stuart and Lieberman (1993) provide healthcare professionals with the mnemonic **BATHE**, for eliciting the psychological context of the client's presenting problem:

> **B** ackground
> **A** ffect
> **T** rouble
> **H** andling
> **E** mpathy

To assess the *background* of the problem, a question such as, "What is going on in your life?," elicits the context of the client's visit. *Affect* can be assessed by asking, "How do you feel about what's going on?" or "What is your mood?" for it allows the client to label his current feeling state. The question, "What about the situation *troubles* you the most?" helps both the healthcare professional and client to focus and may bring out the symbolic significance of the problem or illness. It is also important to assess how the client is *handling* the problem, for it will give an assessment of functioning and provides direction for intervention. Finally, offering *empathy* to the client legitimizes their feelings and provides psychological support.

Carillo, Green and Bentacourt (1999) propose the mnemonic **ESFT**:

> **E** xplanatory model of illness
> **S** ocial factors
> **F** ears and concerns
> **T** herapeutic contract

The healthcare professional first elicits the clients *explanatory model of his/her illness* by asking the client what they believe is causing the problem. This is followed by an assessment of such *social factors* as who cooks, who drives in the family, and can the client get the prescribed medication. *Fears and concerns* are assessed, using the

Tuskegee Study as a metaphor. Finally, a *therapeutic contract* is developed in partnership with the client.

Berlin and Fowkes (1982) suggest the mnemonic, **LEARN,** in conducting a cultural assessment. This mnemonic represents the following 5 steps:

L isten
E xplain
A cknowledge
R ecommend
N egotiate

The first step is to *listen* to the client's perception of their presenting problem. The healthcare professional then *explains* their perception of the client's problem, whether it is physiological, psychological, spiritual, or cultural. The next step is to *acknowledge* the similarities and differences between the two perceptions. At times it is easier for the healthcare professional to acknowledge cultural differences, than to acknowledge and focus on the similarities that they have in common. In order to provide a culturally relevant treatment regimen, it is important to recognize differences, but build on similarities. The third step focuses on *recommendations*, which must involve the client. Finally, the healthcare professional is to *negotiate* a treatment plan, considering that it is beneficial to incorporate selected aspects of the client's culture in providing culturally competent care.

Levine, Like, and Gottlieb (2000) put forward still another mnemonic tool –
ETHNIC. ETHNIC represents the components of:

E xplanation
T reatment
H ealers
N egotiate
I ntervention
C ollaboration

Using this mnemonic model, the healthcare professional is to begin by having the client *explain* their problem. Similar to Kleinman's (1980) explanatory model, the healthcare professional is trying to elicit the client's explanation of the problem. If the client cannot offer an explanation, ask what most concerns them about their problem. It is also important to ask the client what kinds of *treatments* they have tried for their problem. This may include the use of vitamins, herbs and home remedies. Next, the healthcare professional is to assess if the client has sought advice from alternative or folk *healers*, friends, or other individuals who are not healthcare professionals. The healthcare professional then *negotiates*, in an attempt to find an option that will be mutually acceptable to both healthcare professional and client. The healthcare professional determines an *intervention*, which may incorporate alternate treatments. It is important to *collaborate* with the client, family members, other healthcare professionals, healers and community resources during all phases of the assessment.

Dobbie, Medrano, Tysinger and Olney (2003) recommend the **BELIEF** instrument as a cultural interviewing tool. This instrument is based on the LEARN and ETHNIC models. The mnemonic BELIEF represents:

> **B** eliefs
> **E** xplanation
> **L** earn
> **I** mpact
> **E** mpathy
> **F** eelings

The healthcare professional first elicits the health *beliefs* of the client by asking the question, "What caused your illness/problem?" The healthcare professional then obtains an *explanation* of the client's problem by asking the question, "Why did it happen at this time?" It is also important to *learn* more about the client's presenting problem and asking the question, " Help me understand your belief/opinion?," will accomplish this task. By asking the question, "How is this illness/problem impacting your life?," will allow the healthcare professional to assess the *impact* of the client's presenting problem. In addition, the healthcare professional must exhibit *empathy* when interviewing the client and statements such as, "This must be very difficult for you," can convey the feeling of empathy. Finally, it is important to assess how the client is *feeling* about the presenting problem.

Kagawa-Singer and Kassim-Lakha (2003) advocate the **RISK** model as a strategy to reduce cross-cultural communication and increase the likelihood of improving health outcomes. RISK (Reduction Assessment to Ascertain Level of Cultural Influence) represents:

> **R** esources
> **I** dentity
> **S** kills
> **K** nowledge

These authors assert that one way to provide culturally responsive care is to conduct a reduction assessment to elicit information about the client's *resources, identity, skills* and *knowledge*, which will reduce the potential of miscommunication and misdiagnosis. In this model, healthcare professionals must assess tangible *resources* for patients and families, by asking questions such as, "What kind of assistance is available to you in your community that might be helpful?," or "Do you know others in your community who have faced similar difficulties?" Questions also must be asked about the client's individual *identity* and acculturation/assimilation to assess the degree of integration within the ethnic community. Healthcare professionals must familiarize themselves with the actual ability and *skills* of the client and family to navigate the healthcare system and cope with the demands of the disease, itself. Finally, it is important to assess specific

knowledge about the client's health beliefs, values, practices and cultural communication

etiquette.

Like (2004) offers the **ADHERE** mnemonic model as a tool for improving

patient adherence with therapeutic regimens:

A cknowledge
D iscuss
H andle
E valuate
R ecommend
E mpower

The healthcare professional *acknowledges* the need for treatment with the patient and

inquires about prior treatments that have been used. Together, they decide on mutual

goals and desired outcomes of treatment. The healthcare professional then *discusses*

possible and actual treatment strategies, in addition to discussing the consequences of

non-treatment. This discussion can include issues such as treatment efficacy and

prognosis. Patient adherence also involves the *handling* of questions or fears the patient

may express about treatment. These concerns may include issues such as side effects and

length of treatment. The healthcare professional then *evaluates* the patient's health

literacy in order to assess barriers and facilitators to adherence. Finally, the healthcare

professional *recommends* treatment and reviews the treatment plan with the patient. The

healthcare professional *empowers* the patient by obtaining the patient's commitment and

readiness to follow through with the therapeutic regime.

Culturally-Based Physical Assessments

As earlier stated in the definition of cultural skill, healthcare professionals also need to develop cultural skill when performing a physical assessment on culturally diverse clients. The healthcare professional should know how a client's physical, biological and physiological variations influence the ability to conduct an accurate and appropriate physical evaluation (Purnell, 1998; Bloch, 1983).

In performing a culturally-based physical assessment, Bloch (1983) encourages healthcare professionals to internally ask such questions as: "Does the client have ethnic variations in anatomical characteristics?" (e.g., many Vietnamese children are commonly small by American standards, not fitting the published growth curves); "Does ethnic-anatomical characteristics affect physical evaluations?"; "Are there distinct growth and developmental characteristics that vary with a client's ethnic background?" and "How does skin color variation influence assessment of skin color changes and its relationship to the disease process?"

As healthcare professionals we tend to have more of a eurocentric, rather than melanocentric, approach to skin assessmemt. Methododically we are taught that yellow signals jaundice and can be a distinct sign of a liver disorder; pink and blue skin changes are associated with pulmonary disease; ashen or gray color signals cardiac disease; copper skin tone indicates Addison's disease; and the nonblanchable erythema response in patients with a Stage I pressure ulcer (Salcido, 2002, p. 100). However, skin pigmentation of African American clients, and other clients with darker skin, may change the presentation of many common skin manifestations such as pallor, localized hyper-pigmentation lesions, petechiae, erythema, jaundice and ecchymosis.

Inflammation is often missed in clients with dark skin and may not be diagnosed until the flare becomes severe. Palpation must be used in localizing warmth, induration, and tightness of the skin in early cases. Lesions of Karposi's sacoma and Basillary angiomatosis can be overlooked and confused with other lesions in dark-skinned clients (McNeil et al., 2002). A well-lighted examination with palpation of all suspected lesions is important in these clients.

Assessing jaundice in Asian clients is more easily determined by assessing sclera, the palm of their hands and the soles of their feet, rather than relying on the change in skin color. Parreno's (1977) Skin Color Scale for Assessing Normal Skin Pigmentation in Asians is a useful tool when conducting physical assessments on Asians. In striving towards a melanocentric approach to assessing the skin of culturally diverse patients, Purnell and Paulanka (2003) offer the following guidelines for assessing skin variations: 1) establish a baseline color (ask a family member); 2) use direct sunlight if possible; 3) observe areas with the least amount of pigment; 4) palpate for rashes; and 5) compare skin in corresponding areas.

Cyanosis and blood oxygenation levels may present differently in dark-skinned clients than in light-skinned clients. For example, some dark-skinned clients from the Mediterranean region may have very blue lips, which may give a false impression of cyanosis. When assessing anemia in dark-skinned clients, an examination of the oral mucosa and capillary refill at the nail bed may be necessary to obtain an accurate assessment (Purnell & Paulanka, 2003).

The literature clearly documents that we are not doing an adequate job of detecting and reducing pressure ulcers in patients with darkly pigmented skin (Salcido,

2002). Researchers are testing a variety of devices that could be used to detect and diagnose, regardless of skin color, alterations in blood flow and other changes that are specific to ischemia and reperfusion injury associated with the development of chronic wounds (Salcido, p. 100). These technologies include visible and near-infrared spectroscopy, pulse oximetry, laser Doppler, and ultrasound (Sowa et al., 2002; Matas et al., 2001). Salcido adds "that combining such physiologic measures with other clinical information would allow skin and wound care professionals a high degree of sensitivity and specificity in preventing, diagnosing, and treating impending chronic wounds in patients with any skin color" (p. 100).

Skill Acquisition

Conducting a cultural assessment is more than selecting a tool and asking the client questions listed on the tool, it requires cultural skill. The healthcare professional's approach must be done in a culturally sensitive manner. Buchwald et al. (1994) suggest several techniques for eliciting cultural content from the client in a sensitive manner. It is suggested that healthcare professionals listen with interest and remain non-judgmental about what they hear. For example, an African American family may openly tell the healthcare professional they use physical punishment to discipline their children. The African American family's focus on physical forms of discipline may initially present controversial and ethical concerns for the healthcare professional (Campinha-Bacote & Ferguson, 1991). However, the healthcare professional must remain non-judgmental and not assume that child abuse is occurring within the family system. It is important to conduct a culturally sensitive assessment to assess for child abuse. The healthcare professional may find out that this form of discipline is characteristic of a functional and appropriate disciplinary behavior of these caring African American parents. As stated by McGoldrick (1982), strict discipline is a way in which some African American parents protect their children from severe consequences of acting-out behavior.

Healthcare professionals can use other techniques in eliciting cultural information in a culturally sensitive manner. For example, the healthcare professional may want to develop alternative styles of inquiry by adopting a less direct and more conversational approach to assessing the client's background. Healthcare professionals may consider a conversational remark such as; "Tell me about yourself and your family." Another technique is to frame questions in the context of other clients or the client's family. For example, a healthcare professional can say, "I know another client who had such and such an idea of what was wrong. Do you think that?" or "What does your mother think is causing your problem?" Attributing explanations to another person can help clients disclose health beliefs and practices that they may feel initially uncomfortable expressing (Buchwald et al., 1994).

Although there are several techniques available to assist healthcare professionals in eliciting cultural information in a culturally sensitive manner, the healthcare professional may still feel awkward in obtaining this information. This feeling is not unusual, for in learning how to conduct a cultural assessment healthcare professionals pass through several levels of skill acquisition. The Dreyfus Model is a helpful framework for understanding the levels of skill acquisition when conducting a cultural assessment (Dreyfus & Dreyfus, 1980). Although Stuart Dreyfus and Hubert Dreyfus developed their model of skill acquisition based upon their study of chess players and airline pilots, Benner (1984) has applied the Dreyfus Model of skill acquisition to nursing. This model of skill acquisition can be further expanded and used as a framework for assessing healthcare professional's proficiency level in conducting a cultural assessment.

The Dreyfus Model (1980) asserts that individuals pass through five levels of proficiency in skill acquisition: *novice, advanced beginner, competent, proficient, and expert.* The *novice* healthcare professional has little understanding of how to conduct a cultural assessment. They possess the "know that" knowledge but not the "know how" knowledge. They "know that" a cultural assessment should be done on each client, but do not "know how" to conduct it in an effective manner. The *advanced beginner* demonstrates marginally acceptable performance in conducting a cultural assessment and has dealt with enough real situations to recognize meaningful components of the assessment. The novice and advanced beginner take in little of the situation and primarily focus on the rules they were taught when conducting a cultural assessment. The third level of skill acquisition is competence. The *competent* healthcare professional usually has two or three years of experience of conducting cultural assessments with culturally diverse populations. This healthcare professional recognizes what information is to be considered most important and what information is to be ignored. However, the competent healthcare professional lacks the speed and flexibility of the proficient healthcare professional. The *proficient* healthcare professional has worked three to five years with culturally diverse clients. They perceive the information gained from the cultural assessment in a holistic manner, rather than in terms of specific aspects of the presenting problem. At this level of skill acquisition, the healthcare professional is able to hone in on accurate areas of the client's problem in regard to cultural implications.

Finally, the *expert* healthcare professional does not rely on specific rules to gain information from the client. This healthcare professional has an enormous background of experience with culturally diverse populations and has developed an intuitive grasp of how to conduct a cultural assessment in an effective manner. They are able to listen to the client and obtain relevant information. When asked by colleagues why they may ask a question in a particular way, the expert healthcare professional may remark, "Because it feels right."

Summary

In assessing patients it is important to recognize that every patient needs a cultural assessment, not just patients who "look like" they need one (Campinha-Bacote, 1998). Everyone has values, beliefs and practices that influence healthcare practices – it is not limited to ethnic or racial groups. It is just as important to conduct a cultural assessment with Mr. Robert Smith, a European American patient, as it is to conduct a cultural assessment with Mrs. Maria Lopez, who self- identifies as being Mexican. Many times, healthcare professionals use the last name of the patient or the patient's physical appearance as a justification to conduct a cultural assessment. This is offensive, for the basic premise of a cultural assessment is that patients have a right to have their values, beliefs and practices understood, respected and incorporated into their care (Leininger, 1978). This includes *all* patients.

Data obtained from a cultural assessment will allow healthcare professionals to formulate a mutually acceptable and culturally relevant treatment plan. This assessment data will also prevent possible misdiagnosis of the client's behavior. However, to acquire a skill level of expert when conducting a cultural assessment, it is necessary to have many cultural encounters.

CHAPTER 6

Cultural Encounters

"Interestingly, loving care does not require twice the time,
but it does require more than twice the presence."
Erie Chapman

Cultural encounter is the act of directly interacting with clients from culturally diverse backgrounds. The goals of cultural encounters are to generate a wide variety of responses and to send and receive both verbal and nonverbal communication accurately and appropriately in each culturally different context (adapted from Sue et al., 1982). Ting-Toomey (1999) contends that effective cultural encounters should consist of "mindful intercultural communications" and argues that the opposite of mindful cross-cultural communication is "mindless stereotyping"--closed-ended, exaggerated over-generalizations of a group of people based on little or no external validity.

Interacting directly with clients from diverse cultural groups will refine or modify one's existing beliefs about a cultural group and prevent stereotyping. "Culture is elastic - knowing the cultural norms of a given group does not predict the behavior of a member of that group, who may not conform to norms for individual or contextual reasons" (LeBaron, 2003). Healthcare professionals must be cautious and recognize that by interacting with three or four members from a specific ethnic group, does not make one an expert on that group. It is possible that these three or four individuals may or may not truly represent the stated beliefs, values, and practices of the specific cultural group that the healthcare professional has encountered. Therefore, classifications such as "Puerto

71

Ricans think this way," or "Christians prefer that…," have limited use, and can lead to error if not checked with experience (LeBaron, 2003).

Every encounter should be considered a cultural encounter. Healthcare professionals themselves can be viewed as a cultural group with unique values, beliefs, practices and language. Some explicit rules from the American healthcare professional culture may be quite foreign to clients of other cultures. Dube', Goldman, and Monroe (1998) give the following examples:

- Clients must make appointments to be seen.
- Clients see a healthcare professional when they are not sick (well visits for preventive care).
- Clients must disrobe and wear a gown or a drape.
- Healthcare professionals must be credentialed.

Linguistic Competence

Language differences amplify cultural differences, further complicating communication between the patient and healthcare professional. Therefore, cultural encounters require linguistic competence. The National Center for Cultural Competence (Goode & Jones, 2006) defines linguistic competence as "the capacity of an organization and its personnel to communicate effectively, and convey information in a manner that is easily understood by diverse audiences including persons of limited English proficiency, those who have low literacy skills or are not literate, and individuals with disabilities."

Determining the patient's language preference for both spoken and written communication as well as assessing for limited-English proficiency are among the first steps in the process of linguistic competence. Goode and Jones (2006) suggest the following resources to support linguistic competence:

• bilingual/bicultural or multilingual/multicultural staff;

- cultural brokers;
- cross-cultural communication approaches;
- sign language interpretation services;
- multilingual telecommunication services;
- printed material in easy to read, low literary, picture and symbol formats;
- foreign language interpretation;
- materials in alternative formats (e.g. audiotape, Braille, enlarged print);
- TTY and other assistive devices;
- materials tested for specific cultural ethnic and linguistic group; and
- computer assisted real time translation (CART) or viable real time transcriptions (VRT);

The use of linguistic support services, such as interpretation services, must be carefully evaluated. For example, the use of untrained interpreters, friends or family members may pose a problem due to their lack of knowledge regarding medical terminology and disease entities. This situation is heightened when children are used as interpreters. One glaring example is noted in the case of the obstetrical healthcare professional that needed to communicate to her client that she was going to deliver a stillbirth. The healthcare professional did not speak Spanish and used the client's 6-year-old daughter to interpret to the mother that the baby was dead. We can clearly see in this tragic case that a trained medical interpreter was needed. In response to such tragic cases, the United States Office of Civil Rights and Office of Minority Health have taken action. In 1998, The Office of Civil Rights issued a National Guidance Memorandum regarding the care of clients who have limited English proficiency and provided guidance on working with medical interpreters.

When language issues pose a challenge for the healthcare professional, the services of a medical interpreter are advisable. Like (2000) suggests that the mnemonic **TRANSLATE** be used as a guiding framework when working with medical interpreters:

T rust
R oles
A dvocacy
N on-judgmental attitude
S etting
L anguage
A ccuracy
T ime
E thical issues

Like developed this model based on the works of Kraufert and Putsh (1997). This mnemonic addresses the issues of *trust, roles, advocacy, non-judgmental attitude, setting, language, accuracy, time* and *ethical issues.* The healthcare professional must address how *trust* will be developed in the client-interpreter relationship as well as in the relationship with the client's family and other healthcare professionals. The role or *roles* that the medical interpreter will play in the clinical care process must also be considered. For example, will the interpreter serve as a language interpreter, culture broker/informant, culture broker/ interpreter of biomedical culture, or as an advocate? *Advocacy* issues include asking such questions as, "How will advocacy and support for the client and family care occur?" and "How will power and loyalty issues be handled?" The healthcare professional should also consider how a *non-judgmental attitude* will be maintained during this clinical encounter and how his/her personal attitude, values beliefs and biases are to be dealt with. The *setting* is important and the healthcare professional needs to be apprised of where and how the medical interpretation will occur during health care. The healthcare professional must also address *language* issues by asking how linguistic appropriateness and competence will be assessed; how knowledge and information will be exchanged in an *accurate*, thorough, and complete manner; how *time* will be managed; and how confidentiality and other *ethical* issues will be handled during this encounter.

Health Literacy

Linguistic competency requires healthcare professionals to respond effectively to the health literacy needs of populations served. Healthy People 2010 define health literacy as "The degree to which individuals have the capacity to obtain, process, and understand basic health information and services needed to make appropriate health decisions" (cited in Nielsen-Bohlman et al., 2004). Research demonstrates that literacy is the single best predictor of health status - a stronger predictor than age, income, employment status, education level, or racial and ethnic group. Low health literacy has serious consequences for patient outcomes and is fundamental in efforts to reduce health disparities.

According to the 2003 National Assessment of Adult Literacy (NAAL), almost 45% of the United States population (or 93 million Americans) have basic or below basic literacy skills (low literarcy) (cited in The Partnership for Clear Health Communication, n.d.). Low health literacy affects several cultural and ethnic groups including the elderly (66% of United States adults aged 60 and over have either inadequate or marginal literacy skills); impoverished (45% of all functionally illiterate adults live in poverty); minorities (50% of Hispanics, 40% of African Americans, and 33% of Asians have literacy problems); and immigrants (non native English speakers are more likely to have difficulty reading) (cited in The Partnership for Clear Health Communication, n.d.).

The Partnership for Clear Health Communication (n.d.) has developed a solution-based initiative entitled *Ask Me 3* [TM]. *Ask Me 3* [TM] is a tool designed to improve health communication between patients and providers by promoting the following three

questions: 1) What is my main problem?; 2) What do I need to do?; and 3) Why is it

important for me to do this? (The Partnership for Clear Health Communication, n.d.).

Mnemonic Models for Cultural Encounters

Mnemonic models can provide healthcare professionals with helpful guidelines

and suggestions for effective cultural encounters. Clark, Hewson and Fry (1996) suggest

the mnemonic, **PEARLS**, as a framework for cultural encounters with clients. PEARLS

represents the culturally sensitive communication skills of *partnership, empathy,*

apology, respect, legitimization and *support.* Healthcare professionals may want to

incorporate the following suggested comments into their cultural encounters to reflect

what these authors call, "PEARLS of Communication:"

> **P** artnership: "Let's tackle this together."
> **E** mpathy: "That sounds difficult."
> **A** pologize: "I apologize for the wait."
> **R** espect: "Help me understand."
> **L** egitimization: "I hear you."
> **S** upport: "Here is my card, please call if..."

The Boston University Residency Training Program in Internal Medicine,

Diversity Curriculum Taskforce (Bigby, 2003, p. 20) proposes the **RESPECT** model as a

culturally responsive approach during cross-cultural encounters:

> **R** espect
> **E** xplanatory model
> **S** ocio-cutural context
> **P** ower differential
> **E** mpathy
> **C** oncerns
> **T** herapeutic alliance

Healthcare professionals are to enter into the cultural encounter with an attitude of *respect*, both verbally and nonverbally, to the patient. The healthcare professional inquires about the patient's *explanatory model* by exploring the assumptions and beliefs of the patient. In addition to inquiring about the patient's explanatory model, information, from a *socio-cultural context* is also gathered. This includes collecting data regarding the patient's race, ethnicity, class, gender, sexual orientation, immigration status, family and gender roles, and assess how these factors affect care. The healthcare professional is encouraged to acknowledge and pursue the *power* differential in the clinician-patient encounter and relationship. The healthcare professional demonstrates *empathy* by validating the significance of any concerns or fears of the patient, so he/she can feel understood. Eliciting *concerns* or fears of the patient, fosters trust and develops a therapeutic alliance. A *therapeutic alliance* is necessary in order to enhance engagement in, and adherence to, health care recommendations.

Carballeria (1996) recommends the **LIVE & LEARN** model as a framework for practicing cultural competency. Each letter in this mnemonic represents an attitude, activity or strategy to be used by healthcare professionals to create positive encounters with their clients. **LIVE** is the affective component:

L ike
I nquire
V isit
E xperience

If the healthcare professional does not genuinely *like* or appreciate a population, it will be difficult to understand clients who are members of that population. Healthcare professionals need to *inquire* about different cultural groups by familiarizing themselves with the demographics, history, traditions, beliefs, social norms, family structures, strategies for discipline, and preferred forms of address of the populations with whom they work. Knowledge of resources is also important. Carballeria (1996) suggests adopting the attitude of a *visitor* when interacting with those from different cultures. This will assist the healthcare professional to access the client's world and enables the healthcare professional to take cues from the client instead of acting from his/her own worldview. When healthcare professionals perceive themselves as guests, it is natural to be observant and respectful and to emulate social norms. Carballeria also encourages healthcare professionals to *experience* what their client's experience. For example, if your client does not have a car and takes a bus to get to their appointment, the healthcare professional may want to personally take a bus ride as a way of getting to an appointment. This will allow the healthcare professional to experience the many challenges that their clients may have experienced.

LEARN is the strategy component of Carballeria's (1996) LIVE & LEARN model:

L isten
E ssential Cultural Orientations
A cknowledge
R ecommend
N egotiate

Using this framework, the healthcare professional first *listens* for the communication style as well as the content of what is being communicated by the client. Identification of the specific beliefs, values and attitudes of the client (*essential cultural orientation-ECO*), are then pursued by the healthcare professional. The healthcare professional then *acknowledges* the similarities and differences between their culture and the client's culture. While matching the communication style of the client, the healthcare professional is to make *recommendations* by describing the full range of options available and their potential consequences. The healthcare professional should inquire about the client's preferences to acknowledge that the client has a choice. It is important to come to a mutual agreement about the course of action, by *negotiating* an intervention that is acceptable to the client.

Cultural Conflict and Compassion

Although mnemonics can provide healthcare professionals with helpful guidelines and suggestions to avoid potential conflict during the cultural encounter, conflict is inevitable. Culture is always a factor in conflict, whether it plays a major role or influences it subtly (LeBaron, 2003). LeBaron adds "for any conflict that touches us where it matters, where we make meaning and hold our identities, there is always a cultural component." Ironically, conflict can provide healthcare professionals with an excellent opportunity for developing compassion – the emotional task of sharing in one's suffering. Mason Cooley (n.d.) reminds us that "compassion brings us to a stop, and for a moment we rise above ourselves."

Compassion is an emotion of shared suffering and the desire to alleviate or reduce such suffering as well as demonstrating kindness to those who suffer. It is creating a space where patients who suffer can tell their story to someone who can listen with real attention (Nouwen, 1998). As quoted by Maya Angelou (n.d.), "There is no greater agony than bearing an untold story inside you." Compassion is difficult because it necessitates that we enter into the pain of another (Chapman, 2005). When cross-cultural conflict arises, the goal is to respond with compassion. However, the obvious question is, "How does one cultivate compassion in the midst of cross-cultural conflict?"

Arai (cited in Gallaher, 2007) offers the following analogy regarding the relationship between conflict and compassion: "How are rocks polished? You put them in a tumbler, they hit against each other, the sharp edges are knocked off resulting in *mutually polished stones.* The key term here is *mutually.*" Cultivating compassion requires that we understand from the other's point of view and engage in self-reflection of how our actions are affecting the other person (Gallaher). Gallaher adds that "understanding the point of view of the other means you are more likely to respond with compassion rather than judgment." During this reflection process one gradually comes into the awareness that we share more similarities than differences. Our sharp edges have been knocked off resulting in "polished hearts" (Gallaher).

Rolf Kerr powerfully states, "Don't fear mistakes --- fear only the absence of creative, constructive and corrective responses to these mistakes" (cited in Covey, 1989, p. 106). We will all make mistakes and experience degrees of cultural conflict during patient encounters. Probing for the cultural dimension to these conflicts is the key to a successful resolution (LeBaron, 2003). CountryWatch (2001) suggests the following strategies to manage cutural coflicts when they occur:

- Find advantages or a way of connecting to the other person's position so they feel heard.
- Resist looking at everything from your own definition of what is "rational," "logical" and "scientific."
- Recognize that communication obstacles are culturally controlled and often out of one's normal awareness.
- Remember to look for signs of the obstacles in yourself.
- Be aware of different interpretations of what is being said and done.
- Be attentive to personal tension and psychological defenses and develop a plan to address this issue.
- Be alert of the natural tendency to judge and evaluate.

"Sacred Encounters"

Compassion will lead healthcare professionals into a place of meeting in which there is "deep respect for differences and equally intentional openness to the possibility of connection" (Howard, 2003). This connection embodies an encounter, which Chapman (2005) calls "Sacred Encounters." Sacred Encounters occur "whenever we meet another's deep need with a loving response" (Chapman, p. 58). More simply put, it is the merging of love and need. Consider the following scenario:

> A patient is crying out with unimaginable pain. His cry seems to signal not only physical pain but fear, loneliness, and sadness all in one. The nurses are barred from giving further relief medication because of the delicate nature of the patient's condition. Instead, they simply stand by him and stroke his arm and hold his hand and struggle to soothe him with the soft instruments of their voices. They seem like two mothers trying to calm a crying baby – except that this is a full-grown man in exquisite pain. Still, one of them even refers to him as "baby," reinforcing how clearly she understands this patient's deep need for the loving comfort of a mother (Chapman, p. 138).

The intellectual virtues of attentiveness and understanding are needed qualities during Sacred Encounters. Although communicating during cultural encounters consists of two processes: speaking and listening, many healthcare professionals lack the skill of attentive listening. Healthcare professionals must learn to listen responsively or *ting* (the Chinese word for "listening" and connotes attending closely with one's "ears, eyes, and a focused heart") to the sounds, tones, gestures, movements, non- verbal nuances, pauses, and silence in a given situation (Ting-Toomey, 1999). Attentiveness will allow the healthcare professional to focus directly on the client, who is attempting to communicate their feelings. It will result in a better understanding of the client's issues and concerns and in turn the client will feel understood, respected and supported.

Chapman (2005) argues that "loving care does not require twice the time, but it does require more than twice the presence." However, to be fully present with the client, one must be sufficiently involved emotionally (van Hooft, 1999). During cultural encounters, healthcare professionals may experience some uncomfortable emotions as their clients share stories of how it feels to be a minority and of their personal experiences with racism, injustice, and misdiagnosis. These emotions can result in the virtues of, temperance, patience, and compassion.

Non Face-To-Face Encounters

Spoken language is strongly based on face-to-face encounters. Most of the information we receive in face-to-face encounters does not come directly from the words themselves. We use a wide variety of non-verbal cues, such as facial gestures and body movements, to communicate with one another. It has often been said that people "talk" with their eyes and body (LeBaron, 2003). However, not all cultural encounters will be face-to-face interactions.

Telephonic communication has become a cost-effective way of providing health care services to clients. Verbal communication via the telephone elicits challenges for healthcare professionals that are not experienced in non-face-to-face cross-cultural encounters. The healthcare professional must rely solely on verbal communication, without the advantage of relating this verbal communication to the cultural context of the client's non-verbal behavior. This poses a concern for clients who engage in high-context communication in which non-verbal communication plays a central role in the encounter.

High-context and low-context communication refers to the degree to which we rely on factors other than direct speech to convey our messages. It is common for individuals to engage in both high-context and low-context communication. "There are times we 'say what we mean, and mean what we say,' leaving little to be 'read in' to the explicit message (low-context communication) and other times, we send nonverbal cues that we want to have conveyed but do not speak" (LeBaron, 2003). Low and high-context communication may also be useful in understanding specific cultural groups. Healthcare professionals telephonically communicating with a client, who communicates from a high-context perspective, can clearly see how receiving correct communication becomes a major issue in the encounter. Resources, such as "Ear-to-Ear Encounters: A Checklist for Culturally Responsive Telephonic Communication" (Campinha-Bacote, 2003) have been developed to assist healthcare professionals in identifying skills needed for effective telephonic communication and other non-face-to-face encounters.

In addition to telephonic encounters, healthcare professionals may be facing other forms of non-face-to-face cultural encounters. Technology has created such cultural encounters as the Internet, World Wide Web and E-mail communication. Human communication is difficult to capture electronically and we attempt to compensate for this deficit by **bolding our words,** CAPITALIZING OUR WORDS, adding graphics such as a smiley picture ☺, or creating symbols from punctuation marks :-) to convey feelings beyond the written word. These technological encounters, and other non-face-to-face encounters, will continue to challenge healthcare professionals as they develop culturally responsive approaches to health care.

Summary

Successful encounters require healthcare professionals to engage in an ongoing process of honing and applying skills for self-awareness as well as recognizing the unique perspective each patient brings to the clinical encounter (Hunt, 2001, pp. 3-4). Every encounter is a cultural counter and our goal is to make each cultural encounter a sacred encounter. As movingly expressed by Howard (2005),

> ". . . encounter one another in the clear reflection
> of shared honesty, eyes wide open to both our infinite
> oneness as well as our equally unfathomable difference.
> Both sides of the rhetorical polarity are true. At times I
> can know you and connect with you in such deep
> commonality that it may seem as though there is no
> difference between us as we swim together in the flow
> of our human beingness. Yet, at other times, if I am
> awake and conscious of you in your full reality, I am
> pierced by the knowledge of your profound and absolute
> difference from me, your impenetrable otherness, which I
> can never fully know and certainly never be."

Cultural Competency in Healthcare Delivery: "Have I 'ASKED' Myself The Right Questions?"

"Questions are the creative acts of intelligence."
Frank Kingdom

It is important to realize that cultural competency addresses many faces of diversity, for cultural competence goes beyond knowing the values, beliefs, practices and customs of ethnic groups such as African Americans, Asians, Hispanics/Latinos, Native Americans/Alaskan Natives, and Pacific Islanders (Campinha-Bacote, 2003d). As stated early on in this book, in addition to racial classification and national origin, there are many other faces of cultural diversity. Religious affiliation, language, physical size, gender, sexual orientation, age, disability (both physical and mental), political orientation, socio-economic status, occupational status and geographical location are but a few of the faces of diversity. In meeting the needs of these many faces of cultural diversity, healthcare professionals must realize that these faces share a common goal – to obtain quality healthcare services that are culturally responsive and culturally relevant to their specific cultural group.

The Process of Cultural Competence in the Delivery of Healthcare Services model provides healthcare professionals with a model of practice to render culturally competent and culturally responsive health care to *all* clients. In clinically applying this practice model of cultural competence, consider the following question: "In caring for my patients, have I *"ASKED"* myself the right questions?" The below mnemonic, *ASKED,* represents Campinha-Bacote's (2002) self-examination questions regarding the healthcare professional's personal awareness, skill, knowledge, encounters, and desire:

"Cultural Competency in Healthcare Delivery: Have I *'ASKED'* Myself The Right Questions?" ©

Awareness: Am I aware of my biases and prejudices towards other cultural groups, as well as the existence of racism and other "isms" in healthcare?

Skill: Do I have the skill of conducting a cultural assessment in a sensitive manner?

Knowledge: Am I knowledgeable about the worldviews of different cultural and ethnic groups, as well as knowledge in the field of biocultural ecology?

Encounters: Do I seek out face-to-face and other types of sacred encounters with individuals who are different from myself?

Desire: Do I really "want to" become culturally competent?

© Copyrighted by Campinha-Bacote (2002); not to be reprinted without permission

The above **"ASKED"** mnemonic can assist healthcare professionals in informally assessing their level of cultural competence, however, healthcare professionals may want to conduct a more formal self-assessment. The instrument, **Inventory For Assessing**

The Process of Cultural Competence Among Healthcare Professionals - Revised (IAPCC-R) (Appendix C), is a formal self-assessment tool that is based on **The Process of Cultural Competence in the Delivery of Healthcare Services** model and can provide another form of self-assessment. There is also a student version, **Inventory For Assessing The Process of Cultural Competence Among Healthcare Professionals – Student Version (IAPCC-SV)**, of the **IAPCC-R** (Appendix D).

Summary

If you answered each of the five **ASKED** mnemonic questions with a resounding "Yes!" you will have in turn answered the question initially posed in this book, "What does it mean to be a culturally competent healthcare professional?" However, your journey towards cultural competence has only begun. It has been wisely said that it is not the answers to questions that are important; but rather the type of questions one asks. So, I leave you with a second question to ponder - "What will you do to continue your journey towards cultural competence in healthcare delivery?"

Let The Journey Continue!

Brewster, L., van Montfrans, G., and Kleijnen, J. (2004). Systematic review: Antihypertensive drug therapy in Black patients. *Annals of Internal Medicine,* 14(18), 614-27.

Buchwald, D., Caralis, P., Gany, F., Hardt, E., Johnson, T., Mueche, M., and Putsh, R. (1994). Caring for patients in a multicultural society. *Patient Care,* 28(11), 105-123.

Burroughs, V., Maxey, M., and Levy, R. (2002). Racial and ethnic differences in response to medicines: Towards individualized pharmaceutical treatment. *Journal of the National Medical Association,* 94(10), 1-20.

Campinha-Bacote, J. (2006). *Enhancing CARE Through Transcultural Nursing: "Can You Paint With All the Colors of the Wind?"* Presentation at the 32nd Annual Conference of the Transcultural Nursing Society. Annapolis, MD.

Campinha-Bacote. J. (2005a). *A Biblically Based Model of Cultural Competence in the Delivery of Healthcare Services.* Cincinnati, OH: Transcultural C.A.R.E. Associates.

Campinha-Bacote. J. (2005b). A biblically based model of cultural competence. *Journal of Multicultural Nursing & Health,* 11(2),16-22.

Campinha-Bacote, J. (2003a). *The Process of Cultural Competence in the Delivery of Healthcare Services: A Culturally Competent Model of Care* (4th Edition). Cincinnati, OH: Transcultural C.A.R.E. Associates.

Campinha-Bacote, J. (2003b). Cultural desire: The development of a spiritual construct of cultural competence. *Journal of Christian Nursing,* 20(3), 20-22.

Campinha-Bacote, J. (2003c). Cultural desire: The key to unlocking cultural competence. *Journal of Nursing Education,* 42(6), 1-2.

Campinha-Bacote, J. (1998). *The Process of Cultural Competence in the Delivery of Healthcare Services: A Culturally Competent Model of Care* (3rd Edition). Cincinnati, OH: Transcultural C.A.R.E. Associates.

Campinha-Bacote, J. (1996). A culturally competent model of nursing management. *Surgical Services Management,* 2(5), 22-25.

Campinha-Bacote, J. (1995). Transcultural psychiatric nursing: Diagnostic and treatment issues. *Journal of Psychosocial Nursing,* 32(8), 41-46.

Campinha-Bacote, J. (1991). Community mental health services for the underserved: A culturally specific model. *Archives of Psychiatric Nursing,* 5(4), 229-235.

Campinha-Bacote, J., and Ferguson, S. (1991). Cultural considerations in child rearing practices: A transcultural perspective. *Journal of National Black Nurses' Association,* 5(1), 11-17.

Carballeria, N. (1996). The live and learn model for culturally competent family services. Latin American Health Institute, AIA Resource Center, *The Source,* Volume 6, No. 3.

Carillo, J., Green, A., and Betancourt, J. (1999). Cross-cultural primary care: A patient-based approach. *Annals of Internal Medicine,* 130, 829-834.

Chapman, E. (2005). *Radical Loving Care.* Nashville, TN: Baptist Healing Hospital Trust.

Chong, N. (2002). *The Latino patient: A cultural guide for health care providers.* Yarmouth, ME: Intercultural Press.

Clarke, W., Hewson, M. and Fry, M. (1996). *Three Function Card.* [Web site]; accessed 6 Oct. 2004; available from http://www.physicianpatient.org/products.html#publications

Cohen, E., and Goode, T. (1999), revised by Goode, T., and Dunne, C. (2003). *Policy Brief 1: Rationale for Cultural Competence in Primary Care.* Washington, DC: National Center for Cultural Competence, Georgetown University Center for Child and Human Development. [Web site]; accessed 29 April; available from http://www11.georgetown. edu/research/gucchd/ nccc/documents/Policy_Brief_1_2003.pdf

Cooley, M. (n.d.). *Mason Cooley Quotes.* [Web site]; accessed 21 May 2007; available from http://www.brainyquote.com/quotes/authors/m/mason_cooley.html

CountryWatch. (2001). *Cross-Cultural Issues and Information.* [Web site]; accessed 10 April, 2007; available from http://aol.countrywatch.com/aol_ print.asp?v COUNTRY =83& SECTION= APP&TOPIC=CCIAI&TYPE=APPEN

Covey, S. (1989). *The 7 Habits of Highly Effective People.* NY: Simon & Schuster

Cross, T., Bazron, B., Dennis, K., and Isaac, M. (1989). *Toward a Culturally Competent System of Care.* PA: CASSP Technical Assistance Center at Georgetown University Child Development Center.

Culhane-Pera, K. (1996). "The cultural competence continuum." Cited in The Center for Cross-Cultural Health. (1997). *Caring Across Cultures: The Provider's Guide to Cross-Cultural Health Care,* MN: Author.

Cullnan, C. (1999). Vision, privilege and the limits of tolerance. *Electronic Magazine of Multicultural Education,* 1(2). [journal online]; accessed 14 April 2007: available from http://www.eastern.edu/publications/emme/199/spring/cullinan.htm.

DelBello, M., Soutuillo, C., Ochsner, J., et. al (1999). Racial differences in the treatment of adolescents with bipolar disorder. *New Research 379.* Presented at the 152nd Annual Meeting of the American Psychiatric Association, May 18th in Washington, DC.

Diagnostic and Statistical Manual of Mental Disorders: DSM-IV. (1994). Washington, DC: American Psychiatric Association.

Dobbie, A., Medrano, M., Tysinger, J., and Olney, C. (2003). The BELIEF instrument: A preclinical tool to elicit patient's health beliefs. *Family Medicine,* 35(5), 316-9.

Dreyfus, H., and Dreyfus, S. (1980). A five-stage model of the mental activities involved in directed skill acquisition. *Operations Research Center Report,* February 1980.

Dube', C., Goldman, R., and Monroe, A. (1998). "Introduction to Culture and Medical Interactions." In C. Dube', R. Rosen, J. Toohey, et al (Eds.), *Communication Skills for Breast and Cervical Cancer Screening: A Curriculum for Medical Students: Module Three.* Providence, RI: Brown University.

Dubois, C (n.d.). Sacrifice Quotes. *Wisdom Quotes.* [Web site]; accessed 29 April 2007; available from http://www.wisdomquotes.com/cat_sacrifice.html

Eisenberg, D., Davis, R., Etter, L., Appel, S., Wilkey, S., Van Rompay, M., and Kessler, R. (1998). Trends in alternative medicine use in the United States, 1990-1997: Results of a follow-up national survey. *JAMA,* 280 (18), 1569-1575.

Eisenberg, D., Kessler, R., Foster, D., Norlock, F., Calkins, D., and Delbanco, T. (1993). Unconventional medicine in the United States: Prevalence, costs and patterns of use. *New England Journal of Medicine,* 328 (4), 246-252.

Ells, A. (n.d.) "What does the Bible say about. . . Humility?" *Bible.com.* [Website]; accessed 15 April 2007; available from http://www.bible.com/bibleanswers_result.php?id=120.

Fadiman, N. (1997). *The Spirit Catches You and You Fall Down: A Hmong Child, Her American Doctors, and the Collision of Two Cultures.* New York, NY: Farrar, Straus, and Giroux.

Ferdinand, K. (2006). The isosorbide-hydralazine story: Is there a case for race-based cardiovascular medicine? *The Journal of Clinical Hypertension,* 8(3), 156-158.

Fong, C. (1985). Ethnicity and nursing practice. *Topics in Clinical Nursing,* 7(3), 1-10.

Jones, M., Cason, C. and Bond. (2004). Cultural attitudes, knowledge, and skills of a health workforce. *Journal of Transcultural Nursing,* 15(4), 283-290.

Galanti, G. (1991). *Caring for Patients From Different Cultures.* PA: University of Pennsylvania Press.

Gallaher, D. (April 5, 2007). Polishing the Heart. *Journal of Scared Work.* [journal online]; accessed 13 April 2007; available from http://journalofsacredwork.typepad.com/journal_of_sacred_work/2007/04/polishing_the_h.html

Gaw, A. (2001). *The Concise Guide to Cross-cultural Psychiatry.* Washington, D.C.: American Psychiatric Publishing, Inc.

Giger, J., and Davidhizar, R. (2003). *Transcultural Nursing.* St. Louis: Mosby Year Book.

Goode, T. and Jones, W. (2006). *A Definition of Cultural Competence.* Washington, DC: National Center for Cultural Competence.

Harwood, A. (1981). *Ethnicity and Medical Care.* MA: Harvard University Press.

Hassouneh, D. (2006). Anti-racist pedagogy: Challenges faced by faculty of color in predominately white schools of nursing. *Journal of Nursing Education,* 45(7), 255-262.

Howard, G. (2003). Speaking of difference: Reflections on the possibility of culturally competent conversation. *New Horizons for Learning Online Journal,* 9(2). [journal online]; accessed 15 April 2007; available from http://www.newhorizons.org/strategies/multicultural/howard.htm

Hunt, L. (2001). Beyond cultural competence: Applying humility to clinical settings. *Bulletin,* Nov./Dec), Issue 24, pp. 3-4. [journal online]; accessed 13 April 2007; available from http://www.parkridgecenter.org/Page1882.html

Jacobsen, F. (1988). "Ethnocultural Assessment." In L. Comaz-Diaz (Eds.), *Clinical Guidelines in Cross-Cultural Mental Health.* NY: Wiley & Sons.

Jeffreys, M. (2006). *Teaching Cultural Competence in Nursing and Health Care: Inquiry, Action, and Innovation.* NY: Springer Publishing Company.

Kagawa-Singer, M., and Kassim-Lakha. (2003). A strategy to reduce cross-cultural miscommunication and increase the likelihood of improving health outcomes. *Academic Medicine,* 78: 577-587.

Kaufert, J., and Putsch, R. (1997). Communication through interpreters in healthcare: Ethical dilemmas arising from differences in class, culture, language, and power. *Journal of Clinical Ethics,* 8(1), 71-87.

King, M. (n.d.). Cited in Molly Rush's article, "Making Universal Healthcare a Reality."
The Thomas Merton Center. [Web site]; accessed 29 April 2007; available from
http://www.thomasmertoncenter.org/The_New_People/Nov2004/making_universal_healt
hcare_a_re.htm

Kleinman, A. (1980). *Patients and Healers in the Context of Culture*. CA: University of
California Press.

Kleinman, A., Eisenburg, L.M. and Good, B. (1978). Culture, illness and care. *Annals of
Internal Medicine, 88, 251.*

Kudzma, E. (2001). Cultural competence: Cardiovascular medications. *Progress in
Cardiovascular Nursing*, 16(4), 152-160, 169.

Kuno, E. and Rothbard, A. (2004). Racial disparities in antipsychotic patterns for
patients with schizophrenia. *American Journal of Psychiatry,* 159 (4), 567-572.

Lara, G. (June 1997). *Strategies to Improve Health Status for Women of Color.* Paper
presented at the Women of Color Health Conference: Collaborating Today for a Healthy
Tomorrow. Michigan State University, College of Human Medicine in East Lansing,
Michigan.

Lavizzo-Mourey, R. (1996). Cultural competence: Essential measurements of quality for
managed care organizations. *Annals of Internal Medicine*, 124(10), 919-921.

Law, E. (n.d.) *Eric Law.* [Web site]; accessed 31 Jan. 2004; available from http://www.
dioceseofnewark.org/vox1003/vox31003.htm#eric

Law, E. (1993). *The Wolf Shall Dwell With The Lamb.* St. Louis, Missouri: Chalice
Press.

Lawson, W. (1999). *Ethnicity and Treatment of Bipolar Disorder.* Presented at the
152nd Annual Meeting of the American Psychiatric Association on May 19th in
Washington, DC.

LeBaron, M. (2003). "Communication Tools for Understanding Cultural Differences."
Beyond Intractability. Eds. Guy Burgess and Heidi Burgess. Conflict Research
Consortium, University of Colorado, Boulder. [Web site] accessed 10 April; available
from http://www.beyondintractability.org/essay/communication_tools/

Levin, S., Like, R., and Gottlieb, J. (2000). *ETHNIC: A Framework for Culturally
Competent Clinical Practice.* New Brunswick, NJ: Department of Family Medicine,
UMDNJ-Robert Wood Johnson Medical School.

Leff, J. (1981). *Psychiatry Around the Globe.* NY: Marcel Dekker, Inc.

Leininger, M. (1995). *Transcultural Nursing: Theories, Concepts and Practices,* (2nd Ed.) NY: McGraw Hill, Inc.

Leininger, M. (1978). *Transcultural Nursing: Theories, Concepts and Practices.* NY: John Wiley & Sons.

Leininger, M. (1967). The culture concept and its relevance to nursing. *Journal of Nursing Education,* 6(2), 27.
Levy, R. (1993). *Ethnic and Racial Differences in Response to Medication.* VA: National Pharmaceutical Council.

Like, R. (2004). *ADHERE: A Mnemonic For Improving Patient Adherence With Therapeutic Regimes.* From The Providers' Guide to Quality and Culture. [Web site] accessed 10 April 2007 from http://erc.msh.org/quality&culture. Published in Soto-Greene, M., Salas-Lopez, D., Sanchez, J., and Like, R.C. (2004). Antecedents to Effective Treatment of Hypertension in Hispanic Populations. *Clinical Cornerstone,* 6(3): 30-36.

Like, R. (2000). TRANSLATE: For working with medical interpreters. *Patient Care,* 34(9), 188.

Lin, K., Poland, R., and Lesser, I. (1986). Ethnicity and psychopharmacology. *Culture, Medicine, and Psychiatry,* 10, 151-165.

MacIntosh, P. (1989). White privilege: Unpacking the invisible knapsack. *Peace and Freedom,* July/August, 10-12.

Marin, H., and Escobar, J. (2001). Special issues in psychopharmacological management of Hispanic Americans. *Psychopharmacol Bull,* 35 (4): 197-212.

Marsella, A. (2003). Cultural aspects of depressive experience and disorders. In W. J. Lonner, D.L. Dinner, S.A. Hayes, & D. n. Sattler, *Online Readings in Psychology and Culture* (Unit 9, Chapter 4), Center for Cross-Cultural Research, Western Washington University, Bellingham, Washington, USA. [Web site]; accessed 12 April 2007; available from http://www.wwu.edu/~culture

Matas, A., Sowa, M., Taylor, V., Taylor, G., Schattka, B., and Mantsch, H. (2001). Eliminating the issue of skin color in assessment of the blanch response. *Adv Skin Wound Care,* 2001;14:180-8.

May, R. (1975). *The Courage to Create.* NY: Bantam.

McGoldrick, M. (1982). "Normal Families: An Ethnic Perspective." In F. Walsh (Ed.), *Normal Family Process.* NY: Guilford Press.

McNeil, J., Campinha-Bacote, J., and Vample, G. (2002). *BESAFE: National Minority AIDS Education and Training Center Cultural Competency Model.* Washington, DC: Howard Medical School.

Moore, J. (2005). Hypertension: Catching the silent killer. *Nurse Practitioner*, 30(10), 16-18, 23-24, 26-27.

Munoz, C. and Hilgenberg C. (2005). Ethnopharmacology: Understanding how ethnicity can affect drug response is essential to providing culturally competent care. *American Journal of Nursing*, 105(8): 40-48.

Ndura, E (n.d.). The role of cultural competence in the creation of a culture of nonviolence. *Culture of Peace Online Journal*, 2(1) 39-48. [journal online]; accessed 15 April 2007; available from http://www.copoj.ca/pdfs/Elavie.pdf

Neighbors, H. (2003). *The (mis) Diagnosis of African Americans: Implementing DSM Criteria in the Hospital and the Community.* MLK Day Grand Rounds, UM Department of Psychiatry, January 22, 2003. [online]; accessed 27 June; available from http://www.med.umich.edu/psych/mlk2003.htm

New American Standard Bible. (2002). Grand Rapids MI: Zondervan.

Nichols, E. (1987). *Nichols' Model of the Philosophical Aspects of Cultural Difference.* Unpublished paper. Contact: Nichols and Associates, Inc.; 1523 Underwood Street, NW; Washington, DC, 20012.

Nielsen-Bohlman, L., Panzer, A., and Kindig, D. (2004). *Health Literacy: A Prescription to End Confusion.* Washington, DC: National Academies Press. [online]; accessed 29 April 2007; available from http://www.nap.edu/catalog.php? record_id=10883

Nouwen, H. (1998). *Reaching Out.* Grand Rapids MI: Zondervan.

Parreno, H. (1977). "Cultural Health Traditions: Implications for Nursing Care - Oriental Culture." Cited in Orque, M., Bloch, B., and Monroy, L. (1983), *Ethnic Nursing Care.* St. Louis: C.V. Mosby Co.

Partnership for Clear Health Communication. (n.d.) *Ask Me 3* ™ [Web site]; accessed 10 April 10, 2007; available from http://www.askme3.org/

Parreno. H. (1977). "Cultural Health Traditions: Implications for Nursing – Oriental Culture." In M. Orque, B. Bloch & L. Monroy (Eds.), *Ethnic Nursing Care.* St. Louis: C.V. Mosby.

Pedersen, P. (1988). *A Handbook for Multicultural Awareness.* VA: American Association for Counseling and Development.

Pi, E., and Simpson, G. (2005). Psychopharmacology: Cross-cultural psycho-pharmacology: A current clinical perspective. *American Psychiatry Association,* 56 (1), 31-33.

Purnell, L. (1998). "Transcultural Diversity and Health Care." In L. Purnell and B. Paulanka (Eds.), *Transcultural Health Care: A Culturally Competent Approach.* PA: F.A. Davis.

Purnell, L. and Paulanka, B. (1998). *Transcultural Health Care: A Culturally Competent Approach.* PA: F.A. Davis.

Quality Care for Diverse Populations Video. (2007). *American Academy of Family Physicians CME Center.* [Web site]; accessed 29 April 2007; available from http://www.aafp.org/online/en/home/cme/selfstudy/qualitycarevideo.html

Recommendations From the Minnesota Public Health Association's Immigrant Health Task Force. (1996). *Six Steps Towards Cultural Competence.* MN: Author.

Rios-Ells, B., Fritz, N., Duran, A., and Leon. R. (2005). *Be Safe: A cultural competency model for Latinos.* Washington, DC: National Minority AIDS Education and Training Center. [Web site]; accessed 23 April 2007; available from http://www.nmaetc.org/media/ pdf/Be-Safe-Latino.pdf

Rogers, C. (1951). *Client-centered Therapy.* MA: Houghton Mifflin.

Salcido, R. (2002). Finding a window into the skin. *Advances in Skin & Wound Care,* 15(3), 100. [Web site]; accessed 19 April 2007; available from http://findarticles.com/p/articles/ mi_qa3977/is_200205/ai_n9033613

Satel. (2000). *PC, MD: How Political Correctness is Corrupting Medicine.* Washington, DC: AEI Press.

Schaeffeler, E., Eichelbaum, M., Brinkmann, U., Penger, A., Asante-Poku, S., Zanger, U., and Schwab, M. (2001). Frequency of C3435T Polymorphism of MDR1 gene in African people. *Lancet,* 358, 383-384.

Schim, S., Doorenbos, A., Benkert, R. and Miller, J. (2007). Culturally congruent care: Putting the puzzle together. *Journal of Transcultural Nursing* 18(2), 103-110.

Schwartz, R. (2001). Racial profiling in medical research. *New England Journal of Medicine,* 433, 1392-1393.

Smedley, B., Stith, A., and Nelson, A. (2002). *Unequal Treatment: Confronting Racial and Ethnic Disparities in Health Care.* Board on Health Sciences Policy. Institute of Medicine. Washington, DC: National Academic Press.

Snowden, L. (2004). Bias in mental health assessment and intervention: Theory and evidence. *Psychiatric Service*, 93(2), 239-243.

Sowa, M., Matas, A., Schattka, B. and Mantsch, H (2002). Spectroscopic assessment of cutaneous hemodynamics in the presence of high epidermal melanin concentration. *Clin Chim Acta*, 317:203-12.

Sowers, J., Ferdinand, K., Bakris, G., and Douglas, J. (2002). Hypertension-related disease in African Americans. *Postgraduate Medicine*, 112(4). [journal online] accessed 21 Sept. 2006; available from http://www.postgradmed.com/ issues/2002/ 10_02/sowers 1.hn

Stacks, J., Salgado, M. and Holmes, S. (2004). Cultural Competence and social justice: A partnership for change. *Transitions*, 15(3), 4-5. [journal online]; accessed 10 April 2007; available from http://www.advocatesforyouth.org/PUBLICATIONS/ transitions/ transitions1503.pdf

Strakowski, S., McElroy, S., Keck, P., and West, S. (1996). Racial influence on diagnosis in psychotic mania. *Journal of Affective Disorders*, 39(2), 157-162.

Strickland, T., Lin, K., Fu, P., et al. (1995). Comparison of lithium ratio between African-American and Caucasian bipolar patients. *Biological Psychiatry*, 37(5), 325-330.

Stuart, M., and Lieberman, J. (1993). *The Fifteen Minute Hour: Applied Psychotherapy for the Primary Care Physician* (2nd ed.). New York, NY: Praeger.

Sue, D., Bernier, J., Durran, A., Feinburg, L., Pedersen, P., Smith, C., and Vasquez-Nuttall, G. (1982). Cross-cultural counseling competencies. *The Counseling Psychologist*, 19(2), 45-52.

Takeshita, T., Yang, X., Inoue, Y, et al. (2000). Relationship between alcohol drinking, ADH2 and ALDH2 genotypes, and risk for hepatocellar carcinoma in Japanese. *Cancer Letter*, 149(1-2), 69-76.

Tervalon, M., and Murray-Garcia, J. (1998). Cultural humility versus cultural competence: A critical distinction in defining physician-training outcomes in multicultural education. *Journal of Health Care for the Poor and Underserved*, 9(2), 117-125.

The Asthma and Allergy Foundation of America and the National Pharmaceutical Council (2006). *Ethnic Disparities in the Burden and Treatment of Asthma.* Washington, DC: Author. [Web site]; accessed 25 Sept. 2007; available from http://www.npcnow.org/ resources/PDFs/AsthmaEthnicDis05.pdf

Ting-Toomey, S. (1999). *Communicating Across Cultures.* New York: The Guilford Press.

Tylor, E. (1871). *Primitive Culture.* Volume I. London: Bradbury, Evans and Co.
Underwood, S., and Powell, R. (2006). Religion and spirituality: Influence on health/risk behavior and cancer screening behavior of African Americans. *The ABNF Journal,* 17(10), 20-31.

United States Department of Health and Human Services Office of Minority Health. (2007). "Culturally Competent Nursing Models." *Think Cultural Health.* [Web site]; accessed 29 April 2007; available from http://thinkculturalhealth.org/ccnm

U.S. Department of Health and Human Services. (2001). *Mental Health: Culture, Race, and Ethnicity - A Supplement to Mental Health: A Report of the Surgeon General.* Rockville, MD: U.S. Department of Health and Human Services, Substance Abuse and Mental Health Services Administration, Center for Mental Health Services, National Institutes of Health, National Institute of Mental Health.

van Hooft, S. (1999). Acting from the virtue of caring in nursing. *Nursing Ethics,* 6(3), 189-201.

van Ryan, M., and Burke, J. (2000). The effect of patient race and socio-economic status on physicians' perceptions of patients. *Social Science & Medicine,* 50(6), 813-828.

Wandler, K. (2003). Psychopharmacology of patients with eating disorders. *Remuda Review,* 2(1), 1-7.

Wenger, F. (1998). "Cultural Openness, Social Justice, Global Awareness: Promoting Transcultural Nursing With Unity in a Diverse World." In P. Merilainen & K. Vehvilainen-Julkunen (Eds.), *The 23rd Annual Nursing Research Conference 1997: Transcultural Nursing - Global Unifier of Care Facing Diversity With Unity* (pp. 162-168). Kuopio, Finland: Kuopio University Publications.

Whaley, A.L. (1998). Cross-cultural perspective on paranoia: A focus on the black American experience. *Psychiatry Quarterly,* 69(4), 325-343.

Wonders, G. (February 19, 2006). Journey towards wholeness: Cultural competence. *Bradford Community Church Unitarian Universalist: Past Sermons* [Web site]: accessed 19 April 2007; available from http://www.bradforduu.org/pastSermons.asp

Wood, WJ. (1998). *Epistemology: Becoming Intellectually Virtuous.* Downers Grove, IL: InterVarsity Press.

Appendix A
Culturally and Linguistically Appropriate Services (CLAS) in Health Care

CLAS

1. Health care organizations should ensure that patients/consumers receive from all staff members effective understandable, and respectful care that is provided in a manner compatible with their cultural health belief and practices and preferred language.

2. Health care organizations should implement strategies to recruit, retain, and promote at all levels of the organization a diverse staff and leadership that are representative of the demographic characteristic of the service area.

3. Health care organizations should ensure that staff at all levels and across disciplines receive ongoing education and training in culturally and linguistically appropriate service delivery.

4. Health care organizations must offer and provide language assistance services, including bilingual staff and interpreter services, at no cost to each patient/consumer with Limited English proficiency at all points of contact, in a timely manner during all hours of operation.

5. Health care organizations must provide to patients/consumers in their preferred language both verbal and written notices informing them of their rights to receive language assistance services.

6. Health care organizations must assure the competence of language assistance provided to limited English proficient patients/consumers by interpreters and bilingual staff. Family and friends should not be used to provide interpretation services (except on request by the patient/consumer).

7. Health care organizations must make available easily understood patient-related materials and post signage in the languages of the commonly encountered groups and/or groups represented in the service area.

8. Health care organizations should develop, implement, and promote written strategic plans, and management account-ability/oversight mechanisms to provide culturally and linguistically appropriate services.

9. Health care organizations should conduct initial and ongoing organizational self-assessments of CLAS-related activities and are encouraged to integrate cultural and linguistic competence-related measures into their internal audits, performance improvement plans, patient satisfaction assessments, and outcomes-based evaluations.

10. Health care organizations should ensure that data on the individual patient's/consumer's race, ethnicity, and spoken and written language are collected in health records, integrated into the organization's management information systems, and periodically updated.

11. Health care organizations should maintain a current demographic, cultural, and epidemiological profile of the community as well as a needs assessment to accurately plan for and implement services that respond to the cultural and linguistic characteristics of the service area.

12. Health care organizations should develop participatory, collaborative partnerships with communities and utilize a variety of informal and formal mechanisms to facilitate community and patient/consumer involvement in designing and implementing CLAS-related activities.

13. Health care organizations should ensure that conflict and grievance resolution processes are culturally and linguistically sensitive and capable of identifying, preventing, and resolving cross-cultural conflicts or complaints by patients/consumers.

14. Health care organizations are encouraged to regularly make available to the public information about their progress and successful innovations in implementing the CLAS standards and to provide public notice in their communities about the availability of this information.

Source: Assuring Cultural Competence in Health Care: Recommendations for National Standards and an Outcomes-Focused Research Agenda. (2001, March). Retrieved October 17, 2004 from http://www.omhrc.gov/clas/index.htm

Appendix B
Resources in Transcultural Health Care and Cultural Competence

Transcultural Health Care & Cultural Competence

Current Articles (2002-2007)

Agency for Healthcare Research and Quality. (2005). 2005 National Healthcare Disparities Report. Washington, DC: US Department of Health and Human Resources. AHRQ Publication No. 06-0017. December 2005. [Web site]; accessed 7 May 2007; available from http://www.ahrq.gov/qual/nhdr05/nhdr05.pdf

American Journal of Managed Care. (2004). Special issue on health care disparities.

American Journal of Public Health. (2003). Volume 93, Issue, 2. The entire February 1, 2003 issue features a selection of articles on racial/ethnic bias & health.

Anderson, L., Scrimshaw, S., Fullilove, M., Fielding, J., Normand, J., & Task Force on the Community Preventive Services. (2003). Culturally Competent Healthcare Systems. *American Journal of Preventive Medicine*, 24(3S) 68-79.

Andrews, M., Leininger, M., Leuning, C., Ludwig-Beymer, P., Miller, J., Pacquiao, D., and Papadopoulos, R. (2007). *Transcultural Nursing Society Position Statement on Human Rights.* [Web site]; accessed 10 April 2007; available from http://.www.tcns.org

Andrews, M., & Boyle, J. (2003). *Transcultural Concepts in Nursing Care* (4th Edition). Philadelphia: Lippincott, Williams, and Wilkins.

Battle, D. (2002). *Communication Disorders in Multicultural Populations.* Boston: Butterworth-Heinemann.

Berry, E. (2002). Not separate but still unequal: Racial and ethnic disparities in health care. *Clearinghouse Review*, 36, 201-212.

Betancourt, J., Green, A., and Carrillo, E. (2002). Cultural Competence in Health Care: Emerging Frameworks and Practical Approaches. Publication #576. *The Commonwealth Fund.* [Web site]; accessed 7 may 2007; available from www.cmwf.org or at http://www.cmwf.org/usr_doc/betancourt_culturalcompetence_576.pdf

Betancourt, J., Green, A., Carrillo, J., and Park, E. (2005). Cultural competence and Health care disparities: Key perspectives and trends. *Health Affairs*, 24: 499-505.

Bigby, J. (2003). *Cross-cultural Medicine.* Philadelphia, PA: American College of Physicians.

Burroughs, V., Maxey, R., & Levy, R. (2002). Racial and Ethnic Differences in Response to Medicines: Towards Individualized Treatment. *Journal of the National Medical Association,* 94:1-26.

Byrd, W., Clayton, L. (2002). *An American Health Dilemma. Volume 2- Race,* Medicine and Health Care in the United States 1900-2000. NY: Routledge.

Campinha-Bacote, J. (2002). The process of cultural competence in the delivery of healthcare services: A model of care. *Journal of Transcultural Nursing,* 13 (3), 181-184.

Campinha-Bacote, J. (2003). Many faces: Addressing diversity in health care. *Journal of Online Issues in Nursing,* 8(1). [journal online]; accessed 7 May 2007; available from http://nursingworld.org/ojin/topic20/ tpc20_2.htm

Campinha-Bacote, J. (2005). *A Biblically Based Model of Cultural Competence in the Delivery of Healthcare Services.* OH: Transcultural C.A.R.E. Associates.

Chong, N. (2002). *The Latino Patient: A Cultural Guide for Health Care Providers.* ME: Intercultural Press.

Contemporary Nurse. (2003). The Vol. 15 Issue 3, October 2003 of Contemporary Nurse edited by John Daly and Debra Jackson, from the University of Western Sydney is entitled, "Advances in Contemporary Transcultural Cultural Nursing." It is dedicated to Madeleine Leininger and discusses articles on globalization, culture and health, cardiovascular health, and mental health with a particular Australian focus.

Cutilli, C. (2006). Do your patients understand? Providing culturally congruent patient education. *Orthopaedic Nursing,* 25(3), 218-224.

D'Avanzo, C., and Geissler, E. (2003). *Pocket Guide to Cultural Assessment,* 3rd edition. St. Louis: Mosby.

Fortier, J., and Bishop, D. (2004). *Setting the Agenda for Research and Cultural Competence in Health Care: Final Report.* Rockville, MD: US Department of Health and Human Services, Office of Minority Health.

Fletcher, F., Crabtree, A., McKennit, D., Landrie, M., and Magee, P. (2006). *A Systematic Review of the Academic Literature Related to the use and Development of Cultural Competence in Health Promotion and Community Service Professionals.* Edmonton, Alberta: Alberta Cancer Board and University of Alberta.

Galanti, J. (2004). *Caring for Patients From Diverse Cultures.* Philadelphia, PA: University of Pennsylvania Press.

Giger, J., Davidhizar, R., Purnell, L., Harden, J., Phillips, J. and Strickland, O. (2007). American academy of nursing expert panel report: Developing cultural competence to eliminate health disparities in ethnic minorities and other vulnerable populations. *Journal of Transcultural Nursing*, 18(2), 95-102.

Giger, J., and Davidhizar, R. (2003). *Transcultural Nursing* (4th Edition). St. Louis: Mosby Year Book.

Goode, T. and Jones, W. (2006). *A Definition of Cultural Competence.* Washington, DC: National Center for Cultural Competence.

Hasnain-Wynia, R., Pierce, D. and Pittman, M. (2004). *Who, When and How: The Current State of Race, Ethnicity and Primary Language Data Collection in Hospitals.* NY: Commonwealth Fund.

Hassouneh-Phillips, D. and Beckett, A. (2003). An education in racism. *Journal of Nursing Education*, 42(6), 258-265.

Hill, P., Lipson, J. and Meleis, A. (2003). *Caring for Woman Cross-Culturally.* Philadelphia, PA: Davis.

Institute of Medicine (2004). In the Nation's Compelling Interest: Ensuring Diversity in the Health Care Workforce (2004). *The National Academic Press.* Washington, DC: National Academic Press. [Web site]; accessed 7 May 2007; available from http://www.nap.edu/books/ 030909125X/html/

Journal of Transcultural Nursing. (2002). Entire July issue (Volume 13, Issue 3). This issue focuses on the extant models, theories and frameworks of transcultural nursing.

Kai, J. (2003). *Ethnicity, Health and Primary Care.* Oxford: UK University Press.

Kaiser Family Foundation. (2007). *Key Facts: Race, Ethnicity and Medical Care, 2007 Update*, CA: Author:

Kehoe, K. & Melkus, G., Newlin, K. (2003). Cultural Competence Within the Context of Care: An Integrative Review. *Ethnicity & Disease,* 13(3): 344- 353

Leininger, M., and McFarland, M. (2006). *Culture Care Diversity & Universality: A Worldwide Nursing Theory* (2nd.). Massachusetts: Jones and Barlett.

Leininger, M., and McFarland, M. (2002). *Transcultural Nursing: Concepts, Theories, Research & Practice* (3rd ed.). NY: McGraw-Hill Medical Publishing Division.

Leuning, D., Swiggum, P., Wiegert, H., & McCullough-Zander. (2002). Proposed Standards for Transcultural Nursing. *Journal of Transcultural Nursing*, 13(1), 40-46.

Lipson, J., Dibble, S., & Minarik, P. (2005). *Culture and Clinical Care*. CA: UCSF Nursing Press.

Maclean, J., Johnson, M., Rogers, R., and Hoffman, W. (2002). Collecting data on race and ethnicity in managed care: Challenges and suggestions. *JCOM*, 9(5), 259-262.

Morales, L., Puyol, J., and Hays, R. (2003). Improving Patient Satisfaction Surveys to Assess Cultural Competence in Health Care. *California Health Care Foundation*. Oakland, CA: California Health Care Foundation. [Web site]; accessed 29 April 2007; available from http://www.chcf.org/ documents/consumer/PatientSurveysCultural Competence.pdf

McNeil, J., Campinha-Bacote, J., Tapscott, E. & Vample, G. (2002). *BESAFE: National Minority AIDS Education and Training Center Cultural Competency Model*. Washington, DC: Howard University Medical School.

Munoz, C. and Luckman, J. (2005). *Transcultural Communication in Nursing*. NY: Thompson Delmar Learning.

Murphy, S. (2006). Mapping the Literature of Transcultural Nursing. *J Medical Library Association*, 94(2 Suppl): E143–E151.

National Committee on Vital and Health Statistics. (2005). *Eliminating Health Disparities: Strengthening Data on Race, Ethnicity, and Primary Language in the United States*. Author. [online]; accessed 29 April 2007; available from http://www.ncvhs.hhs. gov/ 051107rpt.pdf

Papadopoulous, I., and Lee, S. (2002). Developing culturally competent researchers. *Journal of Advanced Nursing*, 37(3), 258-264.

Policy Research Associates. (2005). *Cultural Competence in Health Care*. Delmar, NY: Author. [online]; accessed 29 April 2007; available from http://bphc.hrsa.gov/hchirc/ pdfs/bibs/28_cultural.pdf

Public Health Reports. (2003). The entire July issue, Vol. 118, Issue 4 is focused on Racial/Ethnic Disparities: Contemporary Issues and Approaches.

Purnell, L., & Paulanka, B. (2003). *Transcultural Health Care: A Culturally Competent Approach* (2nd Edition). PA: F.A. Davis.

Putsch, R. and SenGupta, I., Sampson, A. and Tervalon, M.. (2003). "Reflections on the CLAS Standards: Best Practices, Innovations, and Horizons." *Cross Cultural Health Care Program*. [Web site]; accessed 29 April 2007; available from http://www.xculture.org/research/downloads/CLAS.pdf

Rust, G., Kondwani, K., Martinez, R., Danise, R., Wong, W., Fry-Johnson, Y., Woody, R., Daniels, E., Herbert-Carter, J., Aponte, L. and Strothers, H. (2006). A crash-course in cultural competence. *Ethnicity & Disease,* 16(2), 29-36.

Schim, S., Doorenbos, A., Benkert, R. and Miller, J. (2007). Culturally congruent care: Putting the puzzle together. *Journal of Transcultural Nursing,* 18(2), 103-110.

Satcher, D. and Rubens J. (2006). *Multicultural Medicine and Health Disparities.* McGraw-Hill.

Seibert, P., Stridh-Igo, P., and Zimmerman, C. (2002). A checklist to facilitate cultural awareness and sensitivity. *J.Med.Ethics,* 28 (3): 143-146.

Smedley, B., Stith, A., and Nelson, A. (2002). *Unequal Treatment: Confronting Racial and Ethnic Disparities in Health Care. Board on Health Sciences Policy.* Institute of Medicine. Washington, DC: National Academic Press.

Spector, R. (2004). *Cultural Diversity in Health and Illness.* CT: Appleton-Lange.

Stacks, J., Salgado, M. and Holmes, S. (2004). Cultural competence and social justice: A partnership for change. *Transitions,* 15(3), 4-5. [journal online]; accessed 29 April 2007; available from http://www.advocatesforyouth.org/ PUBLICATIONS/transitions/transitions1503.pdf

Taylor, JS. (2003). Confronting "culture" in medicine's "culture of no culture." *Academic Medicine,* 78(6), 555-559.

Taylor, J. (2003). The story catches you and you fall down: Tragedy, ethnography, and "cultural competence." *Medical Anthropology Quarterly,* 17: 159-181.

Thanasombat, S., and Morris, M. (2006). *Unequal Access to Health Care: A Test Language Services at Alameda County Hospital.* Berkley, CA: The Discrimination Research Center. [online]; accessed 7 May 2007; available from http://drcenter.org/staticdata/Unequal_Access_to_ Health_Care_ DRC.pdf

Wilson-Stronks, A. and Galvez, R. (2007). *Hospitals, Language, and Culture: A Snapshot of the Nation. Joint Commission.* Oakbrook Terrace, IL: Joint Commission.

Wong, P.T.P. (2006). *Handbook of Multicultural Perspectives on Stress and Coping.* NY: Springer.

Yehieli, M. (2005). *Health Matters: A Pocket Guide to Working With Diverse Cultures and Underserved Populations.* Yarmouth, ME: Intercultural Press.

Xu, Y., Shelton, D., Polifroni, E. and Anderson, E. (2006). Advances in conceptualization of cultural competence in nursing: An initial assessment. *Home Health Care Management & Practice,* 18(5), 386-393.

Yuen, F.K.O. (2003). *International Perspectives on Disability Services: The Same But Different.* Binghamton, NY: Haworth Social Work Practice Press.

Websites

Evidenced Based Culturally Competent Care
http://www.usc.edu/hsc/ebnet/Cc/EBCCC.htm

Eastern State University's Office of Cultural Affairs
http://www.etsu.edu/oca/Resources.asp

CLAS Act
http://www.vdh.virginia.gov/ohpp/clasact.asp

ADDM Resource Guide
http://www.amsa.org/addm/ADDM_ResourceGuide.doc

The Provider's Guide to Quality and Culture
http://erc.msh.org/mainpage.cfm?file=1.0.htm&module=provider&language=English

Culturally & Linguistically Appropriate Services National Standards
http://www.omhrc.gov/templates/browse.aspx?lvl=2&lvllD=15

HRSA
http://www.hrsa.gov/culturalcompetence

Cultural Competency Program (CCP)
http://www.med.umich.edu/multicultural/ccp/index.htm

Center for Healthy Families and Culture Diversity
http://www2.umdnj.edu/fmedweb/chfcd/INDEX.HTM

Agency for Healthcare Research and Quality (AHRQ)
http://www.ahcpr.gov/

Office of Minority Health Resource Center
http://www.omhrc.gov

Cultural Competence Resources
http://ublib.buffalo.edu/libraries/units/hsl/resources/guides/culturalcompetence.html

The National Council of La Raza's (NCLR) Institute for Hispanic Health
http://www.nclr.org/

Anti-Racism Resources
http://andromeda.rutgers.edu/~lcrew/antiracism.html

Ethnomed
http://ethnomed.org/

Baylor College of Medicine (BCM) Multicultural Patient Care
http://chronic.bcm.tmc.edu/mpc/home.html

Awesome Library - Multicultural Site
http://www.awesomelibrary.org/Classroom/Social_Studies/Multicultural/Multicultural.html

MEDLINEplus Health Information
http://www.nlm.nih.gov/medlineplus/populationgroups.html

CulturedMed
http://www.sunyit.edu/library/html/culturedmed/

National Center For Cultural Competence (NCCC)
http://www.georgetown.edu/research/gucdc/nccc/

Kaiser Family Foundation - Minority Health
http://www.kff.org/minorityhealth/index.cfm

Cross Cultural Health Care Program (CCHCP)
http://www.xculture.org/

National Multicultural Institute (NMCI)
http://www.nmci.org

Commonwealth Fund (Underserved populations & patient-centered care)
http://www.cmwf.org/index.htm

Health Research & Educational Trust (HRET)
http://www.hretdisparities.org/hretdisparities/html/general/gresources.html

Diversity in Medicine
http://www.amsa.org/div/

Resources for Cross-Cultural Health Care
http://www.diversityrx.org/

Cultural Clues
http://depts.washington.edu/pfes/cultureclues.html

The Center for Cross-Cultural Health
http://www.crosshealth.com/

Multilingual Glossary of Medical Terms
http://allserv.rug.ac.be/~rvdstich/eugloss/welcome.html

Cultural Medicine
http://www.geocities.com/SoHo/Study/8276/CulturalMed.html

Transcultural Nursing Society (TCNS)
http://www.tcns.org

Center For Cross-Cultural Research
http://www.ac.wwu.edu/~culture/

The Access Project
http://www.accessproject.org/

CHISPA Project Information
http://itdc.lbcc.edu/chispa/

The Hmong Health Information Project (Hmong HIP)
http://www.hmonghealth.org

International Cancer Council (ICC)
http://iccnetwork.org/cancerfacts

Walking the Walk: Links to Diversity
http://www.fpg.unc.edu/~walkingthewalk/pages/links.cfm

Think Cultural Health
http://thinkculturalhealth.org/

Program For Multicultural Health Cultural Competency Division
http://www.med.umich.edu/multicultural/ccp/index.htm

The 24 Languages Project:
Consumer Health Brochures in Multiple Languages
http://library.med.utah.edu/24languages/

National Council on Interpreting in Health Care
http://www.ncihc.org/

The Robert Wood Johnson Foundation
http://www.rwjf.org/index.jsp

Visit www.transculturalcare.net
Resources and links are constantly updated

Appendix C
Inventory For Assessing the Process of Cultural Competence
Among Healthcare Professionals – Revised (IAPCC-R©)

Inventory for Assessing the Process of Cultural Competence Among Healthcare Professionals-Revised (IAPCC-R)©

IAPCC-R© is copyrighted by Campinha-Bacote (2002)

Application

The **IAPCC-R**© is designed to measure the level of cultural competence among healthcare professionals. It is specifically intended for the following healthcare clinicians, educators and students: physicians, physician assistants, medical students/residents, licensed practical/ vocational nurses, registered nurses, advanced practice nurses, nursing students, health professions' faculty, dentists, dental students, clinical pharmacists, pharmacy students, physical therapists and physical therapy students. With modifications, it can and has been used to assess other healthcare professionals/students and allied health professions.

Description

The **IAPCC- R**© is a pencil/paper self-assessment tool that measures one's level of cultural competence in healthcare delivery. It consists of 25 items that measure the five cultural constructs of desire, awareness, knowledge, skill and encounters. There are 5 items that address each construct. The **IAPCC-R**© uses a 4-point likert scale reflecting the response categories of strongly agree, agree, disagree, strongly disagree; very aware, aware, somewhat aware, not aware; very knowledgeable, knowledgeable, somewhat knowledgeable, not knowledgeable; very comfortable, comfortable, somewhat comfortable, not comfortable; and very involved, involved, somewhat involved, not involved. Completion time is approximately 10 -15 minutes. Scores range from 25 -100 and indicate whether a healthcare professional is operating at a level of cultural proficiency, cultural competence, cultural awareness or cultural incompetence. Higher scores depict a higher level of cultural competence.

Development of the Instrument

The **IAPCC- R**© is a revision of the Inventory for Assessing the Process of Cultural Competence Among Healthcare Professionals (IAPCC©). The IAPCC© was developed by Campinha-Bacote in 1997 and is based on her model of cultural competence, *The Process of Cultural Competence in the Delivery of Healthcare Services (*1998). The IAPCC© only measured four of the five constructs of this model (cultural awareness, cultural knowledge, cultural skill and cultural encounters) and not the fifth construct of cultural desire. In 2002, Campinha-Bacote revised the IAPCC©, by adding five additional questions to measure the fifth construct of cultural desire. This revision led to the instrument's final name, **IAPCC-R**©.

Obtaining the **IAPCC-R**©

The **IAPCC-R**© is available for review and personal use only by purchasing the book, *"The Process of Cultural Competence in the Delivery of Healthcare Services, 5th Edition* (2007), authored by Campinha-Bacote. There are additional requirements and a fee associated with use of the **IAPCC-R**© beyond a personal self-assessment (see *Permission To Use IAPCC-R*© and *Cost of Using IAPCC-R*©).

Permission To Use **IAPCC-R**©

The **IAPCC-R** © is copyrighted. Formal permission and a fee are required before the tool can be used in a format other than for personal/individual use. To obtain permission to use the **IAPCC- R**©, please mail (no fax/email) your request to Dr. Josepha Campinha-Bacote at 11108 Huntwicke Place, Cincinnati; Ohio 45241. In your request, please include the title of your project, purpose, target population, specific time frame of use, method of administration, study design (i.e. one-time testing or pre/post test design) and a money order (US Dollars only) or check (US Dollars and drawn from a US Bank) for fees associated with your method of administration (see *Cost of Using IAPCC-R* ©). Dr. Campinha-Bacote will return a letter granting permission to use the tool, articulate specific terms regarding use of the tool, and include the number of tools if being used in an onsite pencil/paper format or one copy of the tool if the request is for an offsite administration.

Cost of Using **IAPCC-R**©

There is a fee of $8.00 per tool when administered onsite, in a pencil/paper format for research studies, grants, projects or in any onsite pencil/paper distribution to a group of individuals/participants. In this onsite administration format the **IAPCC-R**© will be hand-distributed to each participant and then personally collected immediately following participants' completion of the **IAPCC-R**©. There is a fee of $20 per tool when administered offsite in such formats as an online secure format for a training program, in-service educational program, academic course, continuing education offering, or when administered in any form of external or internal postal mailing distribution. Please note that the fee is for the number of tools distributed to complete the study; not necessarily the number of participants. For example, if you are conducting a pre/post test design you will need twice the amount of tools as the number of participants. Fees associated with this tool are for a one-time use per aggregate distribution and not for unlimited use. Therefore, permission is required for further use of the **IAPCC-R**© in any additional projects related or unrelated to its initial use.

Reliability

The **IAPCC-R**© has been used extensively within the United States, and reliability was reported from studies conducted in Minnesota, Texas, Nebraska, Pennsylvania, Missouri, New York, Maryland, Washington, New Jersey, North Carolina, Florida, and Massachusetts that yielded an average reliability coefficient Cronbach Alpha of .83. For details of these studies please visit **www.transculturalcare.net/iapcc-r.htm**. The **IAPCC-R**© has also been tested, internationally, in countries such as Portugal, Japan, Finland, Italy, Denmark, Guam, Thailand, Puerto Rico, New Zealand, Ireland, China, Australia, Turkey, England, and South Korea; however, reliability was only reported from studies conducted in Israel, Sweden, South Africa, Taiwan, and Canada, which revealed an average reliability coefficient Cronbach Alpha of .76. For details of these studies please visit **www.transculturalcare.net/iapcc-r.htm**. For more tests of measurement on the **IAPCC-R**© and publications on this instrument please visit **www.transculturalcare.net/iapcc-r.htm**.

Inventory for Assessing the Process of Cultural Competence Among Healthcare Professionals - Revised (IAPCC-R) ©

Copyrighted by Campinha-Bacote (2002)

For self-assessment only; not to be copied or reprinted without permission

Instructions: Read each of the following statements and circle a response

1. Cultural competence mainly refers to one's competency concerning different ethnic groups.

STRONGLY AGREE   AGREE   DISAGREE   STRONGLY DISAGREE

2. I feel that cultural competence is an ongoing process.

STRONGLY AGREE   AGREE   DISAGREE   STRONGLY DISAGREE

3. Factors such as geographical location, gender, religious affiliation, sexual orientation, and occupation are not considered areas of concern when seeking cultural competence.

STRONGLY AGREE   AGREE   DISAGREE   STRONGLY DISAGREE

4. I have a personal commitment to care for clients from ethnically/culturally diverse groups.

STRONGLY AGREE   AGREE   DISAGREE   STRONGLY DISAGREE

5. I feel that there is a relationship between culture and health.

STRONGLY AGREE   AGREE   DISAGREE   STRONGLY DISAGREE

6. I am knowledgeable in the area of ethnic pharmacology.

Very Knowledgeable   Knowledgeable   Somewhat Knowledgeable   Not Knowledgeable

7. I am motivated to care for clients from culturally/ethnically diverse groups.

STRONGLY AGREE   AGREE   DISAGREE   STRONGLY DISAGREE

8. I am knowledgeable about the worldviews, beliefs, practices and/or life ways of at least two cultural groups.

Very Knowledgeable   Knowledgeable   Somewhat Knowledgeable   Not Knowledgeable

9. I am aware of the cultural limitations of existing assessment tools that are used with ethnic groups.

VERY AWARE   AWARE   SOMEWHAT AWARE   NOT AWARE

10. I am knowledgeable in the area of biological variations among different ethnic groups.

Very Knowledgeable   Knowledgeable   Somewhat Knowledgeable   Not Knowledgeable

11. Anatomical and physiological variations do not exist in different ethnic groups.

STRONGLY AGREE   AGREE   DISAGREE   STRONGLY DISAGREE

12. I am aware of specific diseases common among different ethnic groups.

VERY AWARE   AWARE   SOMEWHAT AWARE   NOT AWARE

13. I am willing to learn from others as cultural informants.
STRONGLY AGREE   AGREE   DISAGREE   STRONGLY DISAGREE

14. I seek out education, consultation, and/or training experiences to enhance my understanding and effectiveness with culturally and ethnically diverse clients.
STRONGLY AGREE   AGREE   DISAGREE   STRONGLY DISAGREE

15. I am aware of at least 2 institutional barriers that prevent cultural/ethnic groups from seeking healthcare services.
VERY AWARE   AWARE   SOMEWHAT AWARE   NOT AWARE

16. I recognize the limits of my competence when interacting with culturally/ethnically diverse clients.
STRONGLY AGREE   AGREE   DISAGREE   STRONGLY DISAGREE

17. When my values and beliefs "clash" with my client's values and beliefs I become frustrated.
STRONGLY AGREE   AGREE   DISAGREE   STRONGLY DISAGREE

18. I am aware of some of the stereotyping attitudes, preconceived notions and feelings that I have toward members of other ethnic/cultural groups.
VERY AWARE   AWARE   SOMEWHAT AWARE   NOT AWARE

19. I have a passion for caring for clients from culturally/ethnically diverse groups.
STRONGLY AGREE   AGREE   DISAGREE   STRONGLY DISAGREE

20. I am aware of at least 2 cultural assessment tools to be used when assessing clients in a healthcare setting.
VERY AWARE   AWARE   SOMEWHAT AWARE   NOT AWARE

21. It is more important to conduct a cultural assessment on ethnically diverse clients than with other clients.
STRONGLY AGREE   AGREE   DISAGREE   STRONGLY DISAGREE

22. I feel comfortable in asking questions that relate to the client's ethnic/cultural background.
Very Comfortable   Comfortable   Somewhat Comfortable   Not Comfortable

23. I am involved with cultural/ethnic groups outside of my healthcare setting role.
Very Involved   Involved   Somewhat Involved   Not Involved

24. I believe that one must "want to" become culturally competent if cultural competence is to be achieved.
STRONGLY AGREE   AGREE   DISAGREE   STRONGLY DISAGREE

25. I believe that there are more differences within cultural groups than across cultural groups.
STRONGLY AGREE   AGREE   DISAGREE   STRONGLY DISAGREE

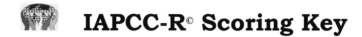

IAPCC-R© Scoring Key

LEVEL OF CULTURAL COMPETENCE:
Culturally Proficient   91 - 100
Culturally Competent   75 - 90
Culturally Aware   51 - 74
Culturally Incompetent   25 - 50

ITEMS # 2, 4, 5, 7, 13, 14, 16, 19, 24, 25
4 pts. = Strongly Agree
3 pts. = Agree
2 pts. = Disagree
1 pt. = Strongly Disagree

ITEMS # 1, 3, 11, 17, 21
4 pts. = Strongly Disagree
3 pts. = Disagree
2 pts. = Agree
1 pt. = Strongly Agree

ITEMS # 6, 8, 10
4 pts. = Very Knowledgeable
3 pts. = Knowledgeable
2 pts. = Somewhat Knowledgeable
1 pt. = Not Knowledgeable

ITEMS # 9, 12, 15, 18, 20
4 pts. = Very Aware
3 pts. = Aware
2 pts. = Somewhat Aware
1 pt. = Not Aware

ITEM # 23
4 pts. = Very Involved
3 pts. = Involved
2 pts. = Somewhat Involved
1 pt. = Not Involved

ITEM #22
4 pts. = Very Comfortable
3 pts. = Comfortable
2 pts. = Somewhat Comfortable
1 pt. = Not Comfortable

Constructs & Reflected Items:
Cultural Awareness: 1, 2, 3, 15, 18
Cultural Knowledge: 6, 8, 10, 11, 12
Cultural Skill: 5, 9, 20, 21, 22,
Cultural Encounters: 14, 16, 17, 23, 25
Cultural Desire: 4, 7, 13, 19, 24

Appendix D

Inventory For Assessing the Process of Cultural Competence
Among Healthcare Professionals – Student Version (IAPCC-SV)

Inventory for Assessing the Process of Cultural Competence Among Healthcare Professionals-Student Version (IAPCC-SV)©

IAPCC-SV is copyrighted by Campinha-Bacote (2007)

Application

The **IAPCC-SV**© is designed to measure the level of cultural competence among students in the health professions. It is specifically intended for the following health professions' students: physician assistant students, medical students/residents, nursing students, dental students, pharmacy students, and physical therapy students. With modifications, the **IAPCC-SV**© can be used with students in the allied health professions.

Description

The **IAPCC-SV**© is a pencil/paper self-assessment tool that measures the level of cultural competence among students. It consists of 20 items that measure the five cultural constructs of desire, awareness, knowledge, skill and encounters. The **IAPCC-SV**© uses a 4-point likert scale reflecting the response categories of strongly agree, agree, disagree, strongly disagree. Completion time is approximately 10 -15 minutes. Scores range from 20- 80 and indicate whether a student is operating at a level of cultural proficiency, cultural competence, cultural awareness or cultural incompetence. Higher scores depict a higher level of cultural competence.

Development of the Instrument

The **IAPCC- SV**© is based on the Inventory for Assessing the Process of Cultural Competence Among Healthcare Professionals-Revised (IAPCC-R©). Researchers using the IAPCC-R© noted that the reliability of this tool was slightly lower when used with students. Vito, Roszkowski, & Wieland (2005) noted in a study of 695 student nurses that the IAPCC-R© could be further revised resulting in a higher reliability of this tool. The **IAPCC- SV**© is a result of modifying the response format of the IAPCC-R© to reflect only responses of strongly agree, agree, disagree, strongly disagree and modifying and deleting selected questions on the IAPCC-R©.

Obtaining the **IAPCC-SV**©

The **IAPCC-SV**© is available for review and personal use only by purchasing the book, *"The Process of Cultural Competence in the Delivery of Healthcare Services, 5th Edition* (2007), authored by Campinha-Bacote. There are additional requirements and a fee associated with use of the **IAPCC-SV**© beyond a personal self-assessment (see *Permission To Use IAPCC-SV© and Cost of Using IAPCC-SV©*).

Permission To Use **IAPCC-SV**©

The **IAPCC-SV**© is copyrighted. Formal permission and a fee are required before the tool can be used in a format other than for personal/individual use. To obtain permission to use the **IAPCC-SV**©, please mail (no fax/email) your request to Dr. Josepha Campinha-Bacote at 11108 Huntwicke Place, Cincinnati; Ohio 45241. In your request, please include the title of your project, purpose, target population, specific time frame of use, method of administration, study design (i.e. one-time testing or pre/post test design) and a money order

(US Dollars only) or check (US Dollars and drawn from a US Bank) for fees associated with your method of administration (see *Cost of Using IAPCC-SV©*). Dr. Campinha-Bacote will return a letter granting permission to use the tool, articulate specific terms regarding use of the tool, and include the number of tools if being used in an onsite pencil/paper format or one copy of the tool if the request is for an offsite administration.

Cost of **IAPCC-SV©**

There is a fee of $8.00 per tool when administered onsite, in a pencil/paper format for research studies, grants, projects or in any onsite pencil/paper distribution to a group of individuals/participants. In this onsite administration format the **IAPCC-SV©** will be hand-distributed to each student and then personally collected immediately following the students' completion of the **IAPCC-SV©**. There is a fee of $20 per tool when administered offsite in such formats as an online secure format for a training program, in-service educational program, academic course, or when administered in any form of external or internal postal mailing distribution. Please note that the fee is for the number of tools distributed to complete the study; not necessarily the number of students. For example, if you are conducting a pre/post test design you will need twice the amount of tools as the number of students. Fees associated with this tool are for a one-time use per aggregate distribution and not for unlimited use. Therefore, permission is required for further use of the **IAPCC-SV©** in any additional projects related or unrelated to its initial use.

Reliability

Fitzgerald, Cronin and Campinha-Bacote (2007) are in the data analysis phase of a study entitled, *Psychometric Testing of a Proposed Student Version of the Tool, "Inventory for Assessing the Process of Cultural Competence Among Healthcare Professionals-Revised"* in which they administered the **IAPCC-SV©** to undergraduate nursing students at Bellarmine University Lansing School of Nursing and Health Sciences to establish reliability of this tool. Please contact Dr. Campinha-Bacote at **meddir@aol** for the results of these findings.

Inventory for Assessing the Process of Cultural Competence Among Healthcare Professionals – Student Version (IAPCC-SV) ©

Instructions: Read each of the following statements and circle a response

1. I believe that cultural competence is a continuous learning process.
STRONGLY AGREE   AGREE   DISAGREE   STRONGLY DISAGREE

2. I have a personal commitment to care for clients from ethnically/culturally diverse backgrounds.
STRONGLY AGREE   AGREE   DISAGREE   STRONGLY DISAGREE

3. I believe that there is a relationship between culture and health.
STRONGLY AGREE   AGREE   DISAGREE   STRONGLY DISAGREE

4. I am knowledgeable about ethnic pharmacology.
STRONGLY AGREE   AGREE   DISAGREE   STRONGLY DISAGREE

5. I am motivated to care for clients from culturally/ethnically diverse groups.
STRONGLY AGREE   AGREE   DISAGREE   STRONGLY DISAGREE

6. I am knowledgeable about the worldviews, beliefs, practices and/or life ways of at least two cultural groups.
STRONGLY AGREE   AGREE   DISAGREE   STRONGLY DISAGREE

7. I am aware of the cultural limitations of existing assessment tools that are used with ethnic groups.
STRONGLY AGREE   AGREE   DISAGREE   STRONGLY DISAGREE

8. I am knowledgeable about biological variations among different ethnic groups.
STRONGLY AGREE   AGREE   DISAGREE   STRONGLY DISAGREE

9. I am knowledgeable of specific diseases common among different ethnic groups.
STRONGLY AGREE   AGREE   DISAGREE   STRONGLY DISAGREE

10. I am willing to learn from others as cultural informants.
STRONGLY AGREE   AGREE   DISAGREE   STRONGLY DISAGREE

11. I seek out education, consultation, and/or training experiences to enhance my understanding and effectiveness with culturally and ethnically diverse clients.
STRONGLY AGREE   AGREE   DISAGREE   STRONGLY DISAGREE

12. I am knowledgeable of at least 2 institutional barriers that prevent cultural/ethnic groups from seeking healthcare services.
STRONGLY AGREE   AGREE   DISAGREE   STRONGLY DISAGREE

13. I recognize the limits of my competence when interacting with culturally/ethnically diverse clients.
STRONGLY AGREE   AGREE   DISAGREE   STRONGLY DISAGREE

14. I become frustrated when my values and beliefs "clash" with my client's values and beliefs.
STRONGLY AGREE   AGREE   DISAGREE   STRONGLY DISAGREE

15. I am aware of some of the stereotyping attitudes, preconceived notions and feelings that I have toward members of other ethnic/cultural groups.
STRONGLY AGREE   AGREE   DISAGREE   STRONGLY DISAGREE

16. I have a passion for caring for clients from culturally/ethnically diverse groups.
STRONGLY AGREE   AGREE   DISAGREE   STRONGLY DISAGREE

17. I am knowledgeable of at least 2 cultural assessment tools to be used when assessing clients in a healthcare setting.
STRONGLY AGREE   AGREE   DISAGREE   STRONGLY DISAGREE

18. I am comfortable in asking questions that relate to the client's ethnic/cultural background.
STRONGLY AGREE   AGREE   DISAGREE   STRONGLY DISAGREE

19. I am involved with cultural/ethnic groups outside of my healthcare setting role.
STRONGLY AGREE   AGREE   DISAGREE   STRONGLY DISAGREE

20. I believe that one must "want to" become culturally competent if cultural competence is to be achieved.
STRONGLY AGREE   AGREE   DISAGREE   STRONGLY DISAGREE

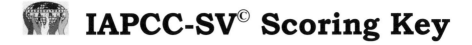

IAPCC-SV© Scoring Key

LEVEL OF CULTURAL COMPETENCE:

Culturally Proficient	75 - 80
Culturally Competent	60 - 74
Culturally Aware	41 - 59
Culturally Incompetent	20 - 40

ITEMS # 1-13 and 15-20
4 pts. = Strongly Agree
3 pts. = Agree
2 pts. = Disagree
1 pt. = Strongly Disagree

ITEMS # 14 (Reverse coding)
4 pts. = Strongly Disagree
3 pts. = Disagree
2 pts. = Agree
1 pt. = Strongly Agree

CONSTRUCTS & REFLECTED ITEMS:

Cultural Awareness:	1, 3, 15,
Cultural Knowledge:	4, 6, 8, 9, 12,
Cultural Skill:	7, 17, 18,
Cultural Encounters:	10, 11, 13, 14, 19,
Cultural Desire:	2, 5, 16, 20

About The Author

Josepha Campinha-Bacote, PhD, MAR, APRN, BC, CNS, CTN, FAAN

Dr. Campinha-Bacote is President and Founder of Transcultural C.A.R.E. Associates, which provides clinical, administrative, research, and educational services related to transcultural health care and mental health issues. She received a B.S. from the University of Rhode Island, M.S. from Texas Women's University, M.A. in Religion from Cincinnati Christian University, and a Ph.D from the University of Virginia. Dr. Campinha-Bacote is Board Certified by the American Nurses Credentialing Center as a Clinical Nurse Specialist in Adult Psychiatric & Mental Health Nursing, credentialed by the Transcultural Nursing Society as a Certified Transcultural Nurse, and holds a Certificate of Authority from the Ohio Board of Nursing to practice as an Advanced Practice Clinical Nurse Specialist. In addition, she holds the academic title of adjunct faculty at several universities and is on faculty at Case Western University in Cleveland, Ohio.

She has been the recipient of several national and international honors and awards, which include the Distinguished Lecturer Award from Sigma Theta Tau International, the 2004 Transcultural Nursing Society (TCNS) Leadership Award, the Ethnic/Racial Minority Fellowship Award from the National Institute of Mental Health, the 2006 Minority Health Knowledge Award from the Ohio Commission on Minority Health and the 2007 University of Rhode Island Distinguished Achievement Award. Dr. Campinha-Bacote is also a Fellow of the American Academy of Nursing and in 2005 was inducted into the TCNS as a Transcultural Nursing Scholar.

Dr. Campinha-Bacote has given more than 1,000 national and international presentations on issues concerning transcultural health care and transcultural psychiatry and has published numerous articles in these specialty areas. She has developed two conceptual models of healthcare delivery, **The Process of Cultural Competence in the Delivery of Healthcare Service** and **A Biblically Based Model of Cultural Competence in the Delivery of Healthcare Services,** which several colleges/schools of nursing, pharmacy, social work, medicine and other allied healthcare disciplines are incorporating into their programs. Based on these models she has developed the instruments, **Inventory for Assessing the Process of Cultural Competence Among Healthcare Professionals – Revised (IAPCC-R), Inventory for Assessing the Process of Cultural Competence Among Healthcare Professionals –Student Version (IAPCC-SV)** and **Inventory For Assessing a Biblical Worldview of Cultural Competence in the Delivery of Healthcare Services (IABWCC).**

In 2000, Dr. Campinha-Bacote served on the National Advisory Committee to the U.S. Department of Health and Human Services Office of Minority Health to develop standards for Culturally and Linguistically Appropriate Services (CLAS) in Health Care. She has also served on the Consensus Building Committee for the development of Culturally Competent Curriculum Modules for Family Physicians and on the National Project Advisory Committee for the Culturally Competent Nursing Modules Project, which were both sponsored by U.S. Department of Health and Human Services Office of Minority Health. In addition, she was a member of the Expert Team for the HRSA/Magna Systems Incorporated contract, "Centers of Excellence Cultural Competence Assessment and Curriculum Development Project. Dr. Campinha-Bacote currently serves as a consultant on several HRSA grants as well as a consultant to several national institutes and centers including the National Center for Cultural Competence (NCCC) in Washington, DC.

Dr. Campinha-Bacote can be contacted by sending an email to **meddir@aol.com** *or visiting her website at* **www.transculturalcare.net**